Industrial Stress Injuries

Industrial Stress Injuries

Larry E. Morris, M.D.

Bourne & Atherton
Los Gatos, California
1989

Industrial Stress Injuries

Published by:
Bourne & Atherton
15950 Cerro Vista
Los Gatos, California 95032

Cover designed by Tech Graphics

Text designed and typeset by Cragmont Publications

Printed by Edwards Brothers, Inc.

Manufactured in the United States of America

Library of Congress Catalog Number 89–92044

ISBN 0-9623609-0-2

Table of Contents

Dedicated to

Dorothea, James, John, Katie, and Peter

Author's Notes

Nearly 25 years as a psychotherapist in different training and practice settings—Vietnam, a Veterans' Administration hospital, The Menninger Hospital, private practice and consulting in the industrial system—have convinced me of a need for full-time clinicians to do more medical writing. The theories of illness and treatment evolve and change, but the patient generally remains the same. *Industrial Stress Injuries* is based largely on clinical material. The lack of systematic and comprehensive treatment of this subject in the literature inspired this text. The most difficult task was to integrate the many dimensions of psychiatric illness when it occurs in industry. Material was drawn from medicine, nursing, psychology, law, workers' compensation, business, rehabilitation, occupational safety, labor relations and government, all of which contribute to the welfare of the injured. Ultimately, however, stress injuries had to be conceptualized from a psychiatrist's viewpoint. For readability purposes, no attempt was made to use both masculine and feminine pronoun forms, and in this book the use of "he" and "his" applies to all members of the work force. The case illustrations are based on actual clinical material derived from thousands of cases. To preserve the privacy of claimants and patients, identifying characteristics, names and settings have been changed. The clinical studies offered are a composite of many cases rather than individual ones. In acknowledgement, I want to express my gratitude to Greg Blanchard for his editing work, and to my wife for the countless hours of assistance in preparing the final text.

Larry Morris

Part I

Dynamic Understanding

CHAPTER ONE

Natural History of Industrial Stress Injuries

For the people who make the everyday decisions about injured workers, it is useful to know that the medical conditions they manage are influenced by a multitude of factors which are not ordinarily encountered in the field of medicine. What sets industrial conditions apart from others is that they become the legally-mandated responsibility of a health care system which is a loose partnership of odd bedfellows, each rooted in self-interest and each having traditional ways of operating. The major parties in the workers' compensation field are claims adjusters, doctors, nurses, lawyers, judges, rehabilitation counselors, psychologists, chiropractors, labor unions, investigators, small business owners, an array of corporate managers, and the occupational medicine departments of large companies. In addition, there are parties who make policy and regulatory decisions about injured workers, such as lawmakers, state agencies, corporate executives, educators, researchers, medical health planners, lobbyists, and the insurance industry. Numerous other vendors and institutions participate in this system.

Depending on the laws, an injured worker is entitled to medical treatment, temporary financial benefits, retraining and other kinds of compensation. In the event of an injury claim, a worker enters a benefit delivery system in which he encounters a seemingly endless array of factors which influence his welfare. The many parties involved in the system cause it to be inefficient, cumbersome and slow to respond to the needs of the injured worker. Sometimes it is unresponsive and highly adversarial. Often, the system seems to have a life of its own, governed primarily by the emotion of fear. Its energies are expended more toward promoting the interests of its various participants, to the neglect of its intended function, which is to restore an injured worker to health and facilitate his return to work. As might be expected, involvement in the system, by itself, commonly leads to a degree of physical and emotional suffering which exceeds that of a worker's original injury. The welfare of the worker is further jeopardized by a *proliferation of variables* at the clinical level when attempts are made to evaluate, treat or retrain him. It is the nature of such systems to increase in complexity whenever one or more parties initiate action. When that happens, the other parties involved in the case must do something to reassess or reestablish their own position. Workers in a compensation system often report feeling as if they were pawns in drawn out chess matches. As the resources of the benefit delivery system are expended at an increasing rate, the more *complicated* the case becomes and the *longer* it remains in the system. Because of these numerous variables, there is a high risk that, at any point, something may go wrong with the case. Even early-on, it can be proposed that the natural history of an industrial stress injury is treatment failure, delayed healing, unexpected disability, excessive frustration and a high incidence of psychiatric complications.

Since these factors have a bearing upon the course of all industrial injuries, the ideas in this book apply equally to primary stress injuries such as post-traumatic stress disorder, and physical injuries such as a low back syndrome. In this book, a stress injury arising secondarily to a physical condition will be understood as a *psychiatric complication.* Making decisions about claimants can be a frustrating and bewildering task. Without thorough knowledge of the many influences in this system, a logical management strategy will elude the professionals in this field. Yet, if the factors which *critically influence* the course of an injury can be identified, and the *particular way* each factor affects the case is known, then industrial stress injuries can be said to have a certain *predictability*. Understanding how injured workers respond to the decisions made about them will enable workers' compensation professionals to make intelligent decisions about the cases they manage. This knowledge will also assist people who make planning decisions about industrial injuries to improve the efficiency and fairness of the benefit delivery system.

This chapter will further develop the concept of the natural history of industrial stress injuries. This will be done by making a *systematic inventory* of the variables which influence industrial stress injuries and the particular way they are expected to affect recovery. These determinants include 1) the industrial and non-industrial elements of a stress injury, 2) the stressors of the compensation system already mentioned, 3) the worker's psychological responses to his injury, 4) secondary gains, 5) treatment conditions, 6) the role of negative bias about psychiatric problems and 7) the distracting effect of false claims of injury.

Chapters Two through Eight will be devoted to an extensive elaboration of these factors. Chapters Nine through Twelve will map out a rational management strategy to help the worker overcome his injuries and return to the work place. The purpose of this study is to identify these determinants early so they can be controlled and recovery kept on course.

ELEMENTS

The two elements of an industrial stress injury are the stressors in the work place and the particular susceptibilities of workers to them. In the industrial system, it is presumed that these two elements are always present, even if the role played by one component is very small or inapparent. An appreciation of the interplay between industrial and non-industrial factors is the first step toward understanding how a worker became emotionally disturbed in the first place and how he might respond to subsequent events or decisions made about his condition. Inevitably, all of us face difficult situations which threaten to disrupt our psychological equilibrium. As individuals, we vary greatly in the ways we respond to such challenges. As a workers' compensation professional, it is useful to know that workers respond to the conditions of the work environment in highly individualistic and predictable ways, according to their strengths, weaknesses, attitudes and a myriad of other psychological and social factors. A job circumstance which is stressful or noxious for one worker might be highly desirable to his coworker. For example, long hours and hard work may cause depression in a low-energy, plodding person who requires frequent breaks from his schedule. But these demands may fulfill the needs of an aggressive person who enjoys perpetual activity and having his resources challenged. Some individuals are susceptible to even the ordinary day to day pressures of employment. For example, an insecure person who requires constant reassurances from his supervisor may feel dejected if his performance is criticized. These remarks would be accepted in stride by a worker who could feel sure of himself without his supervisor's feedback. Similarly, a worker whose feelings of self-worth are contingent upon receiving promotions or raises may feel like a failure if his employer eliminates a desired position to cut costs during a business downturn. This individual doesn't see that the lost promotion is related to economic conditions, and he experiences it personally, as proof of his inadequacy.

The interplay between industrial and non-industrial elements can be illustrated by studying psychological injuries resulting from harassment. It is evident to professionals in the compensation field that there are supervisors who mistreat workers as well as workers who enable this behavior to begin or continue. Close examination of such an injury usually reveals an element of each. Some workers are so sensitive to rude behavior that they feel physically ill if their supervisor has a bad day and takes out his frustrations on the staff. On the other end of the spectrum, some workers are evidently impervious to the gruffest of bosses over a long period of time. An aggressive person will stand up to an intimidating coworker and demand consideration, while a more timid one will enable the harassment to continue.

My examination of Laura, a 30-year-old married college graduate, further highlights these concepts. To supplement her husband's income Laura worked as a receptionist-secretary for a rapidly growing electronics company. Although the salary was not in keeping with her education, Laura loved the stimulation of the job which permitted her to have close contact with interesting people, some of whom were well-known entrepreneurs and scientists in the community. She was very proficient. Visitors often expressed their gratitude to Laura for her considerate treatment, and the company appreciated her diplomatic way of handling people. However, Laura had a minor slip and fall accident at work which resulted in an unexpected period of disability. Months after the incident she was still complaining of aches and pains in almost every part of her body. Her mobility became progressively limited, and she began to miss work. Psychiatric assessment was recommended by Laura's treating orthopedic surgeon when he could find nothing objective to explain her physical complaints.

At first Laura told me she loved every aspect of her job

and denied the presence of stress elements in the office. When we began to talk about it in more detail, however, Laura stumbled on the realization that her experiences with the wife of one of the firm's owners had been very upsetting. Until the interview, Laura had mentally laid aside the memories of this mistreatment. While the owner's wife officially lacked a title, she had free reign to make decisions about the operation of the front office. Organizing it was her contribution to the fledgling company several years before. Rapid growth had made the wife obsolete, but she still showed up at the office every day and involved herself in its operation. She used the foulest imaginable language with Laura and exploded at her for no reason. She could be cruel. Knowing that Laura prized her job, the wife often asked Laura how she might react to being fired. She criticized Laura in the presence of visitors and sometimes threw pencils at her. Not a day went by without Laura finding herself the target of the wife's hostility.

Yet Laura told me that other secretaries were treated as badly, but they fought back. Work in the office was often interrupted by shouting matches between coworkers and the owner's wife. In contrast, Laura never raised her voice. She always tried to be diplomatic. When the wife was around, Laura tried to make herself as "inconspicuous" as possible. This never worked, and the wife seemed to head straight for her. Until the interview, Laura had forgotten that the owner's wife often caused her to leave the office in an agitated state and to walk through the parking lot with tears streaming down her face.

In the evaluation, Laura emerged as a submissive person who was unable to recognize and mobilize angry feelings. She wore a desperate smile to mask her rage. While I think Laura was offended by rude people like anyone else, she pushed her reactive anger out of awareness and never objected. Background history revealed that her father was a military man who ran a regimented household. Laura had vivid memories of her grandmother, a "true lady," who had advised her never to lose her temper and to be polite to others. It had never occurred to Laura that her failure to object to her manager's behavior invited further mistreatment. While Laura's diplomatic ways were well suited to her job dealing with the public, they were self-defeating when it came to remedying the situation with the owner's wife. It was obvious to me that Laura's physical symptoms were an expression of intense emotion which she could neither recognize nor express. Typical of persons who cannot readily perceive their emotional life, Laura experienced mental hurt as physical pain. Becoming physically disabled after a minor slip and fall injury permitted Laura to avoid a noxious work environment, something she couldn't do without her symptoms.

This often-seen industrial scenario was generated by an interplay of industrial and non-industrial elements—Laura's exposure to an intimidating manager and her particular vulnerability to the rude behavior of others. If Laura had not encountered this manager or had possessed ways to defend herself like her coworkers did, the disability from her accident would have been minimal.

For the purpose of studying industrial stress injuries, it is evident from Laura's problems that the industrial and non-industrial elements contributing to them have dissimilar characteristics. Given a certain *stressor* in the work place, there are many different ways in which workers exposed to this condition may respond. Given the known element of an *individual worker*, however, a more predictable reaction pattern to the external environment is expected. This dissimilarity has an important bearing on the strategy of workers' compensation professionals trying to understand these injuries. It may seem natural to think in terms of *cause and effect*, that is, examining the stressor in the work place first and then trying to determine what effect this might have had on the worker. In my experience this leads to a misunderstanding of how psychiatric injuries occur. Rather, it can be seen that psychological injuries arise not so much from cause and effect phenomena, but from multiple factors operating together—*an interaction or interplay.* In the latter scheme, the worker as an individual is a better starting point for study. In analyzing a problem which has multiple variables it is prudent to study first the variable which has the most stable or reliable characteristics. In the industrial system, the most predictive factor is how a certain worker, by virtue of his enduring personality traits and unique life situation, will respond to the ever-changing demands of the job place.

This is an especially useful concept when a worker has a maladaptive character style or what psychiatrists speak of as a personality disorder. In every instance, the background history of such individuals reveals an established pattern of inadequate problem-solving in personal and work areas of functioning. As expected, personality disorders lack the *critical flexibility* needed to cope effectively with change or difficulty at work. As a result, they are especially susceptible to being psychologically injured. For example, a compulsive personality may lack the mental resiliency to adjust to rapid changes in his duties. Assignments requiring him to improvise or change directions on short notice may be overwhelming and lead to depression. A less rigid co-worker may experience the same changes as an expected and normal aspect of his job. Short of a personality disorder, it is the nature of humans to have enduring traits and characteristic ways of dealing with the environment. Our responses are influenced by every aspect of our lives, including our age, genetic endowment, the stage of our life cycle, past experiences, support system of family and friends, education, occupation and cultural background. The circumstances of our life at the time of an accident will strongly influence the way we deal with it. Our pre-existent attitudes about being injured and disabled will have a critical impact on our recovery. Our work ethic, love of job, commitment to our employer and need for an adequate income also determine how we deal with a period of disability. Knowing about the non-industrial element—the worker in the entire context of his life—is so important in understanding stress-related injuries that much of the material in this book will be devoted to this subject.

In addition to responding in an abnormal way to stressors at work and becoming ill in the first place, the worker, now an *injured worker*, may respond maladapatively to the stressful circumstances he faces each step along the way as he recovers. Knowledge of the worker in the total context of his psychological and social existence provides a solid base on which to build an understanding of how he might react when all the other factors which influence his recovery come into play. Predictably, among workers with industrial stress injuries there is an over-representation of persons who have a long-standing history of maladaption in their personal and occupational lives.

HAZARDS OF THE INDUSTRIAL SYSTEM

Perhaps the most important factor determining the quality of the injured worker's recovery is the industrial benefit delivery system. Utilizing its services exposes the worker to hazards which are seldom encountered in other health care fields. As noted earlier, a worker entering the system finds out sooner or later that his welfare is entrusted to a loose partnership of diverse business, professional, bureaucratic and political entities or disciplines, each having a special focus and a limited appreciation for the role played by a fellow partner. The worker learns quickly that the compensation system is governed by the self-interest and fear of these players. It seems to have a life of its own, and the disabled employee discovers that he has little power to influence it. There are times when he cannot tell that he is involved in a health care system. Too much energy is spent to establish the positions of the various parties, and the services he receives in terms of benefits are offered in a perfunctory manner. If he has a psychiatric injury, the worker finds himself misunderstood and even feared, and he senses that no one in the system knows how to manage his injury. He may be discarded as a malingerer or shirker, or he finds his case passed on to the attorneys.

At best, the industrial system is ponderously slow, and too often the benefits are not meted out when the worker needs them. The lack of timeliness may have real traumatizing effects. It is all too evident that delays in diagnosis and treatment will reduce the speed and extent of recovery. Treatment delays for psychiatric conditions will lead to complications such as substance abuse, intractability and suicidal behavior. Excessive frustration is always experienced by a worker involved in this system and may drain the energies he needs to rehabilitate himself. The worker's journey through the compensation system is doubly jeopardized by the fact that while he remains injured or ill, his capacity to cope with external problems is reduced. As long as he depends upon the injury system for help, he is at significant risk for suffering additional insult which may push his recovery onto a destructive course.

At its worst, the benefit system may contribute to psychological and physical damage which greatly exceeds that of the original injury. The critical influence of the industrial system on the course of a worker's condition is that it increases his risks for experiencing treatment failure, prolonged recovery, unexpected disability and psychiatric complications. The numerous hazards to be encountered in the industrial benefit delivery system and the particular ways an injured worker is expected to react to them will be elaborated upon in Chapter Four. There will also be detailed discussion in this chapter regarding how individuals with ineffective problem-solving ability are expected to flounder in such a system.

PSYCHOLOGICAL RESPONSES TO INJURY

Another factor which plays a critical role in the outcome of an industrial injury is the worker's psychological responses to his injury. In terms of losing something highly valued, a serious physical injury may be the most psychologically traumatic event of a person's life. More than just a loss of the intactness of his body or a disruption of his psychological equilibrium, the practical losses stemming from the injury may be disastrous. The worker may lose his career, his goals, his home or his credit. He may suffer a drastic loss of his self-image as an effective and viable human being. People experience their losses in highly individualistic ways. A chronic low back problem, for instance, may be a painful inconvenience to a manager, but it may cause a carpenter to lose his career. An amputation injury may be overwhelming to a young person who had just entered the work market, but it may be accepted philosophically by a worker who is close to retirement. The normal response to such losses is a *grief reaction.* This is a period of mourning which an injured worker must endure in order to adjust psychologically to his losses. Four predictable stages in the grieving process can be identified—denial, anger, depression and resolution. If a worker can effect a successful passage through these stages, he can accept his losses and use his residual assets to achieve a new level of adaptation.

To illustrate the grieving process, consider the commonly-seen responses of a worker who has suffered an injury to a lumbar disc after performing some very heavy lifting. At first he tries to ignore the sensation of something drastic happening in his lower back and his subsequent pain. He tells himself, "It will probably go away," and he finishes the work shift and perhaps comes back to work a few more days as if nothing were wrong. The denial phase is brief, lasting only a few hours and lingering to some extent for a few days. At first, it is too painful for a person to face the reality that he has a problem which may curtail his income and require a long period of treatment and recuperation. However, in a few days, when the pain becomes excruciating and he cannot function, the worker informs his employer of his injury and sees the doctors. Denial quickly gives way to anger, and the injured worker reacts irritably with everyone involved in his case. He thinks that his employer doesn't really believe he has pain, and he experiences the doctors in the emergency room as insensitive to his problem and too busy with other cases. He may resent his employer's inquiries about his health, and during the angry phase he may change doctors. The feelings of shock and resentment which were partially concealed during the first phase come to the surface, and the worker lashes out at everyone. He quarrels with his family and accuses his employer of deliberately allowing him to work in an unsafe environment. During this stage, the injured worker is trying to find an external reason for his psychological anguish.

This phase usually lasts a few weeks. When the intensity of his anger begins to subside, the injured worker becomes more aware of his loss and slowly permits himself to experience the full impact of the back injury on his life. A pervasive sadness sets in, and those around him may notice certain changes such as withdrawal, moodiness, a loss of interest in his favorite activities, tearfulness, a pessimistic attitude and alteration of his eating, sleeping and communication habits. The worker begins to grieve his losses. This is the depressive phase, and it will persist for months. More than in any other period, the worker's energies are directed primarily toward himself. He spends an enormous amount of time preparing himself psychologically to continue his life without the strong back which had served him well in terms of being a valued worker and an effective person.

The stage of resolution begins when the worker sees some light at the end of the tunnel—the possibility that his pain will not last forever and that he may acquire new skills and at some point reenter the work market. The grieving process is coming to an end. The worker emerges from his shell, and those around him notice a renewed interest in previous activities and friends. His depressive symptoms fall away, and his daily activities become more normalized. The worker has accepted the harsh reality that he will be forever different. In grieving, he has made an adequate inventory of his remaining strengths and assets to discover that his life can continue and that happiness may still be forthcoming.

While recuperating, the injured worker normally responds psychologically in other ways. An injury is an emergency condition to humans. It requires that a person's resources be concentrated on the damaged system to promote healing. While a person's resources are thus redirected, some areas of functioning are compromised, especially his ability to deal with demands and pressures from the outside world. Following a serious injury, a worker normally undergoes some measure of psychological regression. He becomes more helpless, and his problem-solving abilities are reduced to more immature, even childlike levels. Demands or problems which were ordinarily handled with ease may be experienced as overwhelming. He may be totally unable to deal successfully with further adversity. For these reasons, an injured worker has a *heightened vulnerability* to further insult or injury. This has a critical bearing on the welfare of the worker as he moves through the benefit delivery system where he is expected to encounter additional stressors.

Grieving and psychological regression are the normal and expected emotional responses experienced by anyone who has suffered a major injury. A worker will normally become more emotionally unstable after an injury than he was before, and his physical distress may even increase. During his recovery, he may feel much worse before he feels better. If the grieving process is uncomplicated, and he is spared further injury or complications, spontaneous resolution of his psychological distress is expected. The normal psychological responses to an injury can be summarized as 1) a grief reaction with stages of denial, anger, depression and resolution, 2) temporary emotional instability, 3) psychological regression, 4) an increased vulnerability to further insult or injury and 5) spontaneous re-equilibration of the psyche.

A failure to grieve and accept losses can result in permanent distortions in a person's psychological equilibrium. Such persons forever carry around the emotional burden of their loss. The pain and shock accompanying their injury never goes away. Energies that would ordinarily be available for constructive involvement in the outside world are drained by inner emotional turmoil. These intense feelings are a permanent part of their emotional make-up. Such persons live constricted, trouble-filled and ungratifying lives. Or they may give up and become psychological invalids.

A more common abnormal psychological response to an injury is an incomplete passage through the grief process. The worker may encounter difficulties and find himself stranded in any of the stages. For reasons which will be discussed in other chapters, an injured worker may become fixated in the angry stage and forever embattle everyone involved in his case or his personal life. His energies are consumed self-destructively by efforts to hold others responsible for his dilemma. Or he may never emerge from the depressive phase. The worker with the deranged back may never see any light at the end of the tunnel and struggle for years with a myriad of depressive and physical symptoms. It may be helpful to the professionals in the industrial system to recognize that much of the emotional turmoil they encounter among injured workers can be explained by a failure to mourn their injuries adequately.

In terms of the natural history of industrial injuries, there is high incidence of abnormal psychological responses, and inevitably a high risk of psychiatric complications. The frustrations and pitfalls of the industrial system interfere with the normal grieving process. They subject an injured worker to additional insults which, because of his increased susceptibility, may result in a separate and distinct stress-induced condition superimposed on the original injury. The occurrence of abnormal psychological responses to injuries and its impact on the course of an injured worker's recovery will be elaborated upon in subsequent chapters.

SECONDARY GAIN

Secondary gain issues play a critical role in the outcome of an industrial injury because they are a total obstacle to the treatment and rehabilitation of the injured worker. This behavior is an attempt, successful or not, to derive a personal benefit that might not be obtainable without a symptom or a disability. This subject is best introduced by clinical material. I identified a critical secondary gain issue during my examination of Ross, a 28 year-old single carpenter who had failed to return to work one year following a relatively minor injury. Ross was referred for evaluation by the industrial carrier because of unexplained neurological symptoms after a falling board glanced off the back of his head. The accident left him dazed and bleeding but not unconscious. The diagnoses of a slight concussion and a scalp laceration were made. No complications were expected, and he was released to work ten days after the accident. However, many months after the accident, Ross complained of dizziness, blurred vision and faintness. He misplaced his tools and forgot how to do simple carpentry procedures. He was unable to hold a job. In familiar public places, he became disoriented, and several times while shopping he collapsed and was taken to an emergency room by ambulance. Friends were afraid to leave him alone, and they wouldn't let him drive. Ross insisted that the blow had damaged his brain, although nothing objective could be found to explain his symptoms. Extensive diagnostic procedures, including a brain scan and neuropsychological testing, revealed no evidence of an organic brain syndrome.

Despite a history of symptoms which were suggestive of an organic brain syndrome, there was no clinical evidence of this problem. The most prominent finding on examination was acute depression, a problem Ross strongly denied having. He also emerged as an immature person who was more reminiscent of young teenager than a young man of 28, which was his chronological age. By way of background history I learned that he was the youngest of six children born to a father who was an upper level manager in a large corporation and a mother who never worked outside the home. The father was seldom involved with Ross but expected him to attend college and become a professional like himself. However, Ross identified more closely with his mother, who indulged him well into his adult years and secretly gave him money. Ross's life style in high school revolved around surfing and the drug scene. With his mother's approval he dropped out of school during his junior year and began to work as a carpenter.

At the age of 22 Ross married. His wife objected to his marijuana smoking and his lack of interest in their infant son, but there had been no major confrontations or separations. During the interview I learned that two weeks before the accident, Ross had returned home from a football game he had attended with his friends to discover a note from his wife indicating she had taken their son and gone to live with her parents. During the first year of the separation, which was also the post-injury period, Ross made numerous attempts to reconcile with his wife, but she refused to meet with him. His friends even felt obligated to keep his wife informed about his health problems, but she showed no interest in returning to the relationship. The only times she responded to Ross were the occasions when he had been brought to a hospital after collapsing in public. While Ross's wife had not yet filed for divorce, a reconciliation seemed unlikely.

From the information I had, it was clear that Ross's injuries were relatively minor and did not prevent him from returning to work as a carpenter. His neurological symptoms and prolonged disability were related to his failed marriage. I was convinced that his way of presenting himself as a brain damaged and helpless person was an attempt to compel his wife to return. As a youngster, Ross easily manipulated his mother whenever he faced difficult or demanding circumstances. Until his wife's departure he had controlled her in the same way, usually getting what he wanted without consideration for his family. While this attempt at reconciliation was unsuccessful, it was perhaps the only means available to a self-centered and immature person like Ross who was accustomed to getting his way with others. It was the only time that someone close to Ross had turned against him.

A reconciliation was the hoped-for secondary gain to be derived from his helplessness. As long as Ross pursued this gain from the accident, efforts to facilitate his return to a productive life would be futile. They would probably have a paradoxical affect, and Ross would get worse rather than better. Being a functional person is unwanted. For Ross, his disability is valuable, and he would act even more helpless if someone tried to assist him. Ross holds his symptoms in ransom to get his family back and will not relinquish his disability until there is a resolution of his dilemma. He would have to work through the loss of his family and perhaps consider that his marital problems are of his own making.

Secondary gain phenomena are commonplace. They may crop up in any human situation which calls for a quick solution to a desperate problem. Additionally, they appear when a frustrated person has a chance opportunity to indulge a long-standing wish or to meet an unfulfilled need. They are expected in a compensation system. An injured worker is privileged both by the status assigned to sick people in our society and the benefits owed by his employer. An accident is an opportunity to claim infirmity, which is used to obtain any of a seemingly endless variety of personal advantages. In addition to manipulating other people as Ross is trying to do, the gains from illness include money, retirement, avoiding an unwanted job or an obnoxious boss, expressing anger or disguising a weakness. In Ross's case, the personal crisis which led to a secondary gain phenomenon occurred *very close in time* to the industrial accident. In other cases, the personal dilemma which gave rise to secondary gain behavior may be a *long-standing* one.

For example, a person who has felt neglected by his spouse or family for many years magnifies his helplessness in order to get attention at home. Or a disfranchised person might prolong his disability to have some entitlement.

Someone who has felt insignificant all of his life takes advantage of an injury to feel important. The special attention he receives from doctors, lawyers, rehabilitation counselors and the court, is worth the price he must pay in terms of being disabled. Secondary gain may enter the clinical picture *after* an industrial injury, when a worker faces a psychological crisis during recuperation. An individual who feels mistreated after an injury may delay recovery to spite his employer. Retaliatory feelings are discharged indirectly by prolonging disability, a secondary gain which can be described as a compensation grudge. Or a worker may unconsciously sabotage his rehabilitation program to disguise the fact that his self-confidence for reentering the work market is badly shattered.

Secondary gain phenomena influence industrial injuries by defeating the efforts of workers' compensation professionals to return injured people to their jobs. Secondary gain phenomena will be discussed in depth in Chapter Five. Also offered in this chapter is a definition which has practical value in industrial cases, along with additional clinical material and early detection.

CONDITIONS OF TREATMENT

A critical determinant for the outcome of a stress injury is the set of conditions under which psychiatric treatment takes place. The benefits of modern medical science cannot be used by patients at the clinical level unless certain ingredients are present. Compared to others, a compensation health care system creates psychotherapy settings which are fundamentally unsound. To begin with, privacy by law is not preserved. With other parties having access to information, there is no safe or stable base for encouraging communication of an individual's most personal and sensitive concerns.

Without this, psychiatric treatment usually doesn't work. A lack of confidentiality would be expected to inhibit the worker from sharing his emotional pain with another. What the patient reveals is contaminated by a realistic concern that his remarks will affect the delivery of his benefits.

In a compensation scheme, the worker cannot control his benefits. Access to diagnostic procedures and treatment is blocked by third and fourth parties. Long delays in performing these fundamental tasks contribute to chronicity, and for many injuries, a lost opportunity for corrective surgery or other remedies. Yet another example of unsound treatment conditions is the absence of a qualified medical manager. The initiation of treatment is less related to the recommendations of physicians than to the plodding operation of a multi-party health care system. By the time psychiatric treatment is authorized, it is often too late to prevent the problem from becoming chronic or evolving into a more debilitating condition. Delays are extremely frustrating to the stress-injured worker, and a secondary gain issue such as a compensation grudge may appear and preclude a favorable outcome.

Psychiatric treatment of stress injuries is undermined by many distractions. Numerous personal setbacks and losses occur when a worker no longer has an adequate income. He may not be able to keep up with bills, send the rent check or make his car payments. He may have to move and in the process disrupt his family or lose his circle of friends. During a long recovery, losses tend to mount, and a worker may lose his financial credit or find himself unable to afford health insurance. With each setback, the worker may react with intense emotion. These distractions repeatedly aggravate his psychiatric condition and severely undermine treatment. Litigation pressures also drain the energies of psychiatric treatment as there are expectations by other parties to break confidentiality and scrutinize every aspect of the worker's being. The failure to answer medical-legal questions quickly invades the therapeutic process, creating distrust or interrupting it altogether.

More than in a non-industrial health care program, the industrial system encourages helpless behavior on the part of the injured worker. By the time a worker enters treatment, he has acquired an unrealistic expectation that the employer must fulfill the obligation to "cure" him without any effort on his part. Psychiatric treatment is misperceived as a remedy which can be utilized in the role of a passive beneficiary. This attitude will preclude an effective treatment, since no one has such powers, and the work of psychotherapists is facilitative, not "curative." Psychiatric treatment rests upon a shared undertaking. Few stress-injured workers are adequately prepared to accept some responsibility for getting well. A compensation system tends to provide services to workers who have few resources to fall back upon, and a large number lack the knowledge or psychological sophistication to utilize these services. Similarly, there is a disproportionate number of people within the system who handle difficulty by acting helpless and depending excessively on others for solutions. Many are not candidates for conventional psychiatric treatment.

Even when some of these obstacles are surmounted, the worker may not be fortunate enough to have a psychotherapist who is familiar with the natural history of industrial stress injuries. The therapist may not appreciate the high incidence of secondary gain behavior or its destructive effect on recovery. He may not realize that treating someone who is not working or otherwise involved with the external world is useless. Or he may not foresee that the pitfalls of the industrial system will reinforce his patient's symptoms. Too often the therapist addresses the wrong issues. For instance, he forgets the fundamental task in treating injuries which is to assist the patient in grieving his losses. He is overly eager to provide solutions and overlooks the growth-giving advantages of a facilitative approach. Doing this encourages helpless behavior more than it does self-sufficiency. The therapist who lacks an intimate understanding of these determinants doesn't see that psychotherapy is often counterproductive in a compensation system.

For all of these reasons, the conditions for treating psychiatric injuries may not be sufficiently optimal for a favorable result. Some hard decisions must be made about initiating or continuing a useless treatment, since this tends to do more harm than good and contributes to a downhill course. Chapter Six will be devoted to an in-depth discussion of why treatment often doesn't work with industrial stress injuries. This chapter will also show how workers with certain kinds of enduring traits are especially difficult to treat.

NEGATIVE BIAS

An attitude of negative bias about psychiatric disorders strongly shapes the course of recovery of the stress-injured worker. The critical role of this attitude is that it leads to decisions about claimants which are based on emotion rather than the merits of the case. Objectivity can be lost while dealing with a psychologically upset person if the ways we are reacting emotionally to him are not taken into account. A person who is struggling with fear, rage, despondency, or other intense emotion may cause us to experience the same feelings.

From time to time all of us have felt like expressing strong emotion. But in the acculturation process we have learned ways to apply restraint and conduct ourselves so that we appear under control. This is especially true if there are expectations for professional and businesslike behavior. Those involved in human service occupations have to deal constantly with a wide variety of needy and demanding clients. To provide services, they must additionally deal with the personalities of their coworkers, supervisors and outside parties. It is never easy to remain poised while interacting with so many different people, and there are times when this is impossible. The last thing wanted on a difficult day is to encounter a client who has lost his controls. Such persons make us feel like we are losing our own. For these reasons, our responses to them can be negative.

Objectivity can also be lost if we encounter a worker who attributes his disability to difficult job conditions which we coped with successfully. Unrecognized resentment causes us to view him as a shirker, a weakling or malingerer. Most people are provoked when their professional efforts are misunderstood by an unreasonable client, and no one likes to be bullied about by an angry one. Psychiatric patients can be difficult, and reacting emotionally to them is normal and expected. When this happens, we are at risk for developing attitudes and making decisions about these persons which increase our emotional comfort and have little to do with the objective evidence. We are at risk for rejecting such persons, passing the buck to others in the industrial system or sweeping the problem under the rug in hopes that it will go away.

Even more commonly, we might adhere to the traditional bias about psychiatric problems which holds that a person can extricate himself from his dilemma by a sheer act of will. In this thinking, a person claiming depression and suicidal urges can turn his symptoms on and off like a faucet. A person with agoraphobia simply doesn't want to feel better and go to work. Such a person, we can argue, is worthy of contempt. Or we might *deny that psychiatric problems exist in the first place.* Claims of emotional distress then are merely the subjective productions of manipulative people who are so different from ourselves they can be considered as alien-like.

Misunderstanding of mental health problems is commonplace, and acceptance of psychiatry as a helping profession is not widespread. A lack of objectivity invariably leads to destructive decision-making. The influence of negative bias of the natural history of stress-induced injuries is that such workers become derailed within the system. They are avoided, neglected and passed on irrationally to others as lacking in credibility. Decisions are made to release the tension felt by the industrial practitioner, and the rehabilitation needs of the worker are left unmet. An attitude of negative bias contributes significantly to a delayed diagnosis, excessive disability and a chronic illness. Chapter Seven will go into more detail on the reasons for biased attitude about mental disorders and offer clinical illustrations.

PSEUDOINDUSTRIAL INJURIES

The factor which most distracts from the task of providing benefits to the stress-injured worker is the need to weed out claims of injury which have no connection to the work place. In this situation, a worker attributes a problem in his personal life, such as an illness or family crisis, to something which happened at work. Since these conditions are falsely blamed on his job, they might be described as *pseudoindustrial stress injuries.* Sorting them out from genuine work injuries consumes much time and energy, and the determination of a worker's eligibility for benefits is often greatly delayed. Here, the adjuster has an nearly impossible task. Benefits claimed for conditions not caused by the work place must be denied. Yet in the sorting-out process he doesn't want to create additional problems for the worker who has a compensable injury. The worker may not be spared this hardship. Before receiving treatment or other benefits, the claimant is stressed by unfamiliar litigation activities and a prolonged period of uncertainty. Most areas of his functioning are placed on hold, and setbacks occur in his personal life. The predictable costs to the worker are the multitude of complications seen in many industrial accidents. The costs to the system are considerable.

Claims of false injury take two forms which are differentiated by the presence or absence of conscious intent. First are claims in which a worker unconsciously displaces a personal problem to an event or circumstance at work. A desperate problem such as a debilitating anxiety disorder or a failed relationship is disconnected from its origins in the worker's personal life and attached irrationally to his job. At least temporarily, the worker has found a way to be upset without having to feel responsible for his distress. The falsely claimed stressor at work becomes a repository for the worker's emerging problem. Detailed analysis of such cases reveals a strong temporal relationship between the "injury" and a desperate personal problem which has come to a head. Commonly more than one problem is found. No link to the alleged job stressor can be discovered, and it is presumed that the claimant's symptoms are entirely attributable to nonwork dilemmas.

The second kind of false claims concern symptoms or a disability which are deliberately produced and offered, and they are presumed to meet the definition of malingering as set forth in DSM-III-R. In a compensation system a high index of suspicion for malingering is kept because of the obvious incentives available such as money and avoidance of responsibility. Yet this condition is elusive and probably underdiagnosed. A definite determination of its presence is hampered by the lack of a single clinically-reliable indicator. Even when incentives are evident and there are no objective findings, a presumptive diagnosis can only be made when there is strong positive evidence. In Chapter Eight there is a detailed inventory of the positive indicators of malingering. The literature on industrial malingering sheds little light on the detection of these distracting conditions, and clinical material was used extensively to study this problem.

■ ■ ■

The natural history of psychiatric problems in industry is determined by the factors outlined in this chapter. Most of them have a negative impact on recovery, and the tendency of stress injuries is to have a poor prognosis. Exerting control over these special influences, however, will permit industrial professionals to reverse this natural tendency and promote a more favorable outcome. The remainder of Part I is devoted to an elaboration of these critically influencing factors.

CHAPTER TWO

Elements of a Psychiatric Injury

The elements of a psychiatric injury are the stressors of the work place and the particular susceptibilities of the worker to them. In a given case, these two elements are always present. We presume this to be true, since only a small number of people exposed to the same stressful situation develop a psychological injury. Even catastrophic events of the kind expected to traumatize anyone, fail to cause an emotional injury in the majority of those so exposed. This phenomena suggests that stress victims have certain vulnerabilities. In clinical practice the elements can usually be identified. Knowledge of human psychobiology is incomplete, and in some cases the contribution of these two elements is not apparent.

Stress-related injuries are difficult to understand. To explain their occurrence, industrial professionals often think in terms of a *cause and effect* mechanism. For instance, the appointment of a more demanding chief executive officer might be viewed as the cause of an upper manager's debilitating anxiety disorder. But this explanation is unsatisfactory when we consider that a dozen of his co-managers handled the change in stride. The development of a psychiatric injury also requires a non-industrial element which is the worker—his personality traits, strengths and weaknesses, his age, education, and all the other aspects of his past life and current functioning. On close analysis of stress cases, an *interplay* of industrial and non-industrial factors can almost always be found. Focusing on how these elements interact with each other is a more useful approach than cause and effect, and it sheds meaningful light on the origins of these perplexing and complicated conditions.

Certain stressors of the work place are familiar enough. Long hours, overwork, deadlines, shift work, noxious coworkers, bullying bosses, sexual harassment, accountability programs, dangerous work conditions and a "bottom line" management mentality all contribute to the stress-related injuries suffered by tens of thousands of workers each year in this country. These disorders have also been linked to more subtle pressures such as job insecurity, monotony, underutilization, an impersonal work environment, "burnout" occupations, ambiguity of assignments and changing work conditions. It is not the purpose of this book to make an inventory of common job stressors and show that they are statistically related to psychiatric injuries. As a matter of practice, compensation professionals make decisions about an individual who has problems. In a given case, statistical data cannot help them sort out the intricacies leading to the worker's disability or map out a helping strategy. In a system where the focus is on one case at a time, intimate knowledge of the individual worker is essential to intelligent decision making and planning. The role of worker's special vulnerabilities is less appreciated than the well-known stressors listed above. The remainder of this chapter will be devoted to a discussion of the predictable ways in which an injured person, by virtue of his enduring behavioral patterns and unique life situation, interacts maladaptively with the stressors of the work place and contributes to his own breakdown.

While both elements are critical, the worker rather than the occupational stress factor, is a better starting point for studying psychiatric injuries. As outlined in Chapter One, this is true because a group of workers exposed to the same stress element at work will react in a *spectrum* of ways, whereas the worker as an individual is generally *predictable* in his way of coping with the outside world. Examining the individual worker in detail will enable an industrial professional to understand why he became psychologically ill in the first place and, more important, help him predict how the injured worker will respond to decisions made about his welfare during recovery.

Some workers have personality traits which are invariably maladaptive in provocative circumstances. As illustrated in Chapter One, Laura's denial of her angry reactions and failure to express them, even minimally, to an intimidating superior unwittingly invited further mistreatment. Workers with passive-aggressive traits mismanage their reactive anger in different ways. Rather than dealing with noxious work elements directly or constructively, passive-aggressive persons discharge their reactive resentment indirectly by underperforming. Managers of these workers become aware of growing tardiness, absenteeism, procrastination, inefficiency, errors or forgetfulness in carrying out assignments. The name of this pervasive trait is derived from the assumption that such an individual is passively expressing covert feelings of aggression or hostility. Falling-down-on-the-job behavior naturally invites an adversarial relationship with supervisors. This conflict becomes self-perpetuating as the worker reacts to deserved criticism with additional occurrences of underperformance. Though of his own making, the resulting tension can be traumatizing to the worker, who eventually may claim disability because of emotional and physical distress.

A worker with more adaptive traits would appreciate his reactive rage as an *honest response* to mistreatment. He would act upon it constructively, discussing his reactions with the offending coworker or opening up administrative channels available in the employment setting for this purpose. By defusing the conflict early-on, the worker better skilled at managing anger can spare himself further psychological turmoil and a full-fledged illness. The same self-defeating scenario occurs when a passive-aggressive person sustains a physical injury. A worker placed on a medical leave because of a toxic exposure, for instance, may prolong his recovery as a way to retaliate for being forced to work in unsafe conditions. Similarly, failing to recover from a fractured ankle may be an indirect way for passive-aggressive worker to mobilize covert resentment about the frustrations he encounters in his treatment or rehabilitation program.

Persons with enduring paranoid traits are more aggressive and direct in their responses to perceived mistreatment. Because of mistrust and pervasive suspiciousness, they tend to interact maladaptively with a wide variety of industrial stressors. Hypersensitive to the slightest insult or criticism, workers with paranoid traits make mountains out of molehills and quickly become antagonistic in the work place. In the event of a stressful job situation or an unwanted assignment, such persons become hostile and near-combative. As might be expected, they are overrepresented in the caseloads of workers' compensation professionals. Paranoid personalities lack an ability to compromise or to cope with the uncertainties, ambiguities or delays commonly encountered in a compensation system. Facilitating their return to work after a physical injury can be an embattling experience. Corporate managers and insurance adjusters describe them as "impossible to deal with," and they report feeling uneasy or frightened while talking with them in person or by telephone. Losing control is a very threatening circumstance to a paranoid personality, and this will likely be his fate when he enters the industrial benefit system. Such individuals do poorly in the system and are prone to developing excessive disability and psychiatric complications.

By way of illustration, I evaluated a young police officer with a cervical strain who became acutely depressed during his recovery. He emerged as a suspicious man who had always reacted defensively to the bantering comments of co-officers. Lacking a sense of humor, and exquisitely sensitive to criticism, the young man lashed out whenever he perceived a challenge to his ability or courage. Paranoid traits often caused him to have defensive confrontations with superiors. Yet, paranoia was evidently a valuable trait while he patrolled the high-crime neighborhoods to which he was assigned, and he had many citations and awards in his personnel file. While on disability, however, the officer resented his employer's routine inquiries about his recovery. He accused the workers' compensation manager of shorting his benefits. He had an angry confrontation with his orthopedic surgeon and changed doctors. While on leave, his department was reorganized, and the officer misconstrued his upcoming reassignment as a "punishment." Depression and smouldering rage led to a breakdown of his relationship with those involved with his care. These conflicts prolonged his recovery. After a long period of disability, the officer was released to his job, but his personality traits continued to be maladaptive.

Within days of returning, he developed a transient emotional breakdown when an older officer badgered him about his restrictions. Attuned to the young man's vulnerabilities, the senior officer never passed up an opportunity to exploit his colleague's weaknesses. When this scenario was played out to its extreme, the victim became immobilized by rage and a recurrence of his neck problems. While others in the department had had their "buttons pushed" by this particular officer, they simply badgered him back. While the young officer's paranoid traits may have been valuable insofar as helping him survive as a patrolman on the streets, they were maladaptive when his career was temporarily interrupted by an injury, and when he was unable to protect himself from the bullying behavior of a coworker. In the first instance, entering the industrial system caused him to lose control over his destiny, a circumstance which is threatening to a paranoid person. In the second, the officer lacked the sense of humor and social savvy needed to deal with a colleague who attacked his vulnerabilities.

Workers with dependency traits are frequently maladaptive in their efforts to cope with industrial stressors. Their special vulnerabilities are well understood by treating psychiatrists who see many in their practices. Indecisive and lacking in self-confidence, such persons avoid independent functioning and become followers in the work place. Keeping a harmonious relationship with others is critical to their feelings of well-being. By means of accommodating and helpless behavior, dependent perishabilities are adept at getting other people to structure their lives. The major decisions about their occupational activities are left to others. Bosses are so impressed by their eagerness to please that they heap extra duties upon these workers or assign them jobs no one else would want. While these people find themselves with more direction than they bargained for, they seldom complain. Their silence in the matter is necessarily interpreted as approval, and dependent people unwittingly invite even more in the way of demands upon their time. Fearful of jeopardizing a relationship, they are reluctant to make demands upon coworkers. Even when a supervisor detects dissatisfaction and asks what kind of a job would be more preferable, a dependent individual backs down at once. Because of the interplay of accommodating behavior and an abundance of unwanted work assignments, these workers commonly struggle for years with pent-up job dissatisfaction. They are highly prone to having depressions, anxiety disorders and psychologically induced physical conditions.

Still others fulfill dependency needs vicariously by choosing careers in which they can be solicitous to needy people. They become nurses or social workers, caring for others in the same way they would unconsciously like to be taken care of themselves. At times, they identify excessively with needy clients or patients and involve themselves beyond the scope of professional services and expected hours of employment. Dependent individuals are vulnerable to developing the "burnout syndrome." A worker in the service-to-people field who possesses more adaptive psychic mechanisms would maintain professional objectivity and not permit himself to be drained by the demands of his clients. He would find ways to meet his psychological needs outside of the work place.

Workers with dependency traits are usually able to function adequately as long as their work environment is well structured, and they have access to tangible proof of acceptance by others. They are fragile and vulnerable. If given decision-making or planning duties, their psychological equilibrium may be thrown out of balance. They are easily upset if external supports are withdrawn, which might happen if they receive a negative performance review or if a boss who has indicated some favoritism toward the worker is replaced by one who is more objective or even "fair."

A more complex problem arising from a dependency conflict involves the mental mechanism of *counterdependency.* Workers with this personality trait are common but often undetected in the case loads of compensation professionals. Such men and women resort to extreme measures (Nemiah, 1978) to avoid knowing about their dependency wishes or revealing them to others. Their lifestyle is shaped by a desperate effort to disguise an unrecognized wish to be taken care of. To this end, they assume behavioral traits which are 180 degrees in the opposite direction. The name of this trait is based on the assumption that their exaggerated independence is an attempt to counter or neutralize traits which are the exact opposite.

Such individuals are fiercely self-sufficient and permit no one to assist them. There is a history of having assumed adult responsibility during childhood or early adolescence, and a lifestyle totally filled with work and commitments. Time is rarely set aside for recreational or personal hobbies. They welcome being the strong person for their friends and coworkers. Much like dependent workers who are eager to please, counterdependent persons are at a high risk for exhausting their physical and psychological resources in the work place. An even more debilitating result may occur if they sustain a major physical injury such as a ruptured lumbar disc requiring surgery. A prolonged period of recuperation forces such a person into the unfamiliar position of depending upon others. A predictable and commonly-seen pattern of increasingly helpless behavior follows.

At first, the worker becomes highly anxious and moody at having to be inactive for the first time in his life. He minimizes the severity of his physical condition and makes it difficult for treating physicians to help him. As the months go by, however, his symptoms unexpectedly become refractory to all forms of medical intervention. At the same time, the counterdependent person becomes increasingly demanding. Long after the back injury has stabilized, the worker remains aggressively dependent upon his family, his doctors and the industrial treatment system. Those around him are often startled by his helpless behavior. During recovery, the worker's behavior has shifted from acting "super-independent" to a position of an equally excessive dependency. At first, pain and disability were caused by a ruptured disc, but now they are prolonged by compelling psychological factors.

As a result of counterdependency, this person was capable of working hard and taking on heavy responsibilities. But this adaptive mechanism lacked flexibility. When put under a severe strain by a disabling injury, it enabled unrecognized dependency needs to be invited into open expression by mandated inactivity and the care-giving behavior of his family and the medical community. After the initial period of protest, such a person can find a way to tolerate *not working* since he can view this as something forced upon him by an industrial accident. In doing so, his self-image as a motivated person is still intact, but he is prevented from being active by circumstances beyond his control, namely pain and disability. After a long period away from the work place, the worker has learned to gratify formerly-denied dependency needs without having to know about them. No longer motivated to return to productive life, this worker has now become a chronic psychological invalid. This condition is superimposed on a physical condition which has since cleared. It has resulted from an interplay of the industrial accident and his counterdependency traits. His personality make-up rendered him susceptible to having a period of inactivity which he learned to enjoy without having to feel guilty.

Workers may be susceptible to an occupational stressor because of the unique circumstances of their current personal lives. A worker who is grieving the loss of a parent may be unable to deal with upheavals taking place in his job. If his company is being taken over by another, he might have to face the loss of a hard-won position or adapt to a different community. These occupational stressors may interact with the trauma of losing a family member and lead to a major depression. A good support system at home enables a worker to tolerate many noxious elements at work. An understanding spouse, healthy children and sympathetic friends provide the psychological strength needed by employees to endure long hours, heavy responsibilities, bullying bosses, drug addicted co-workers or constantly changing duties. Without this kind of support, he is less able to cope with these pressures and is at higher risk for developing a stress-related condition.

Moving to an undesirable neighborhood, a child taking drugs or the departure of a best friend to another community may collapse a support system and make a worker susceptible to injury.

A person's age or the stage of his life cycle also critically influences his way of dealing with industrial stress elements. For example, a person who has only a few years of productivity left may decide to endure an extremely difficult job, while a younger coworker would move on at once. This is illustrated by my experience with Stuart, a 60 year-old district supervisor employed by a professional association. Stuart was a retired Army officer, and this was his second career. He moved up quickly in the organization and earned a reputation for bringing order and quality field services to previously neglected districts. However, there were strong political forces in the operation of the association, and the arrival of a new director led to a widespread shakeout of upper management. To gain control of the association, the new director earmarked many district supervisors, including Stuart, for replacement or retirement. Younger colleagues prudently resigned and sought employment elsewhere.

But as a former infantry officer, Stuart decided to "fight it out." He told me that jobs of this sort would be impossible to find for a man his age, and he wasn't ready to retire. Without the support of the director or anyone else in the organization, however, Stuart couldn't function. He was easily manipulated into taking assignments which were programmed to fail, and the director made life miserable for him. He became the victim of numerous embarrassments and humiliating encounters with association members. At the age of 60, Stuart met failure for the first time in his life. His self-confidence vanished, and he developed a panic disorder which totally immobilized him. Many people in the work force are in Stuart's position. Because of very similar reasons, workers in their fifties and sixties have a special susceptibility to change in the work place.

Another factor which increases a worker's vulnerability to having an industrial psychiatric disorder is being an immigrant. For reasons which are far too numerous to list, a disproportionate number of persons who were born in other countries become victims of industrial stress here. The burden of being a breadwinner is greater for the first-generation than subsequent ones, as they ordinarily face many additional difficulties in their personal and occupational lives. As a matter of necessity, foreign-born workers may have to take work that no one else wants. Entry-level wages require them to work at more than one job. As a result of maximally utilizing their resources, the span of their work lives may be drastically shortened. Obligations to relatives in their country of origin may continue, and they may not enjoy the convenience of an automobile or comfortable living conditions. Commonly, immigrants are forced to enter the work market at a level which is below their accustomed occupational or socioeconomic status. A civil engineer from an Asian country, for instance, may not be able to obtain a state license and may be forced to take employment as an assembler. Or an office manager may have to become a childcare worker because his skills do not meet business standards.

A failure to adjust to different gender role expectations in the United States is a common element in the industrial stress injuries of foreign-born workers. On one occasion I evaluated a young man from a Central American country who located a well-paying job as a corporate accountant. He had no difficulty performing his duties, but within two years developed an adjustment disorder with a work inhibition. In his department, the young man was assigned to a series of female supervisors, the last of whom was demanding and sometimes critical of his work. This was highly threatening to the young man since in his culture the traditional role of women was subservience. Working with females who were equals was anxiety-provoking enough, but being accountable to a woman, especially an outspoken one, was an adjustment he could not make. Supervisors from different cultures must make a similar adaptation. For instance, a male administrator from a Middle Eastern country was expected to supervise an ambitious young female manager who was born in the same country. This was a task he could not perform because of his gender role expectation that women should be devalued. An adversarial relationship led to a harassment claim by the young woman and a demotion for the administrator, who filed a stress claim of his own.

Immigrant workers are at risk for doing poorly once involved in the industrial benefit delivery system. Language and cultural barriers may be insurmountable. Having their lives influenced by a powerful and impersonal bureaucratic system may be terrifying. The system may be incomprehensible to them. Mistrust of adjusters, attorneys and physicians or other industrial professionals is expected. Initial encounters may be so distressing to such workers that avoidant behavior characterizes the course of their recovery. For all of these reasons treatment and rehabilitation may fail, and these workers tend to have prolonged recoveries.

A worker's past life experiences and attitudes about being injured may heighten his vulnerability to certain stressor factors on the job. On one occasion I examined a woman in her forties who accidently splashed acid in her eyes. Within 48 hours the burns to her cornea had healed completely, and no residual visual defect was expected. However, the woman complained of a variety of vague and shifting eye impairments such as pain, blurred vision and an intolerance to sunlight. The outside world was experienced as a place where reinjury was imminent, and she became a housebound invalid. Background history revealed that her grandfather had been blinded by an accident, and as a young girl she had been frightened by the story of his accident which was frequently retold by family members. As a result of this experience, this person had grown up with the misconception that the eye was the most fragile organ in the body and that even trivial injuries would lead to blindness. Many months of psychiatric treatment were necessary before this medical misinformation was corrected and she could be encouraged to resume a normal life and risk going back to a job.

In another case, an early life experience caused a worker to have a very special vulnerability. A married mother trained to become a court stenographer when her youngest child entered school. At first, she had no difficulty with her new occupation. Within two years, however, the stenographer developed severe headaches, nausea, vomiting and a precipitous weight loss. These physical symptoms progressed and threatened to disrupt her career. She filed a claim for physical conditions which she initially attributed to working for a difficult agency and the exacting nature of her work. As the treating psychiatrist, I discovered a temporal relationship between the onset of her symptoms and her assignment to a series of trials involving child molestation. After several months of therapy, the stenographer began to have memories of having been molested herself as a youngster. Until the exposure to testimony concerning child abuse, she had pushed the memories of these traumatic experiences out of awareness. While less dramatic than these two illustrations, most of us have had past experiences which make us emotionally susceptible to certain kinds of job pressures. The self-selection process usually protects us from these elements, and we seek jobs which feel comfortable. However, we cannot always have control over our assignments.

Discovering the two elements of an industrial stress

injury enables a compensation professional to understand its origins. A knowledge of these forces will suggest a management strategy which can be tailored to the worker's unique needs. Without understanding how the work and nonwork elements operated together to cause pathology, there will be no logical way to reverse the processes which produced it. The natural tendency of stress injuries to have a downhill course will prevail, and the recovering worker remains at risk for suffering complications such as delayed healing, unexpected disability and treatment failure. In this chapter emphasis is placed on studying the more predictive element which is the injured worker. A familiarity with the individual in the entire context of his life will explain not only how he was injured, but suggest how he might respond to decisions made about him during recovery.

CHAPTER THREE

Hazards of the Industrial System

The quality of the injured worker's recovery depends upon how the industrial system performs its job. By nature, a compensation system has many pitfalls. The professionals entrusted to deliver its benefits are hampered by complexities and shortcomings rarely seen in other health care fields. Not only are *multiple* services provided—health care, temporary income and retraining—but there are *constraints*. Only those conditions which are attributable to the work place can be treated. A very large number of professional, bureaucratic and business entities participate in the system's operation. Among its major players are doctors, judges, lawyers, claims adjusters, rehabilitation professionals, psychologists, chiropractors, investigators, small business owners, labor union representatives and insurance executives. In the corporate world important decisions about the injured are made by occupational health nurses, personnel specialists, human resource managers, safety engineers and workers' compensation managers. In the background, the employee's welfare is influenced by policy and regulatory entities such as state agencies, lawmakers, educators, lobbyists, medical health planners and the insurance industry. The numerous parties cause the industrial system to be inefficient, awkward and slow to respond to the injured person's needs. Too often it is unresponsive and adversarial. The reasons are easy to understand.

While the system has a self-contained character, few of the players listed above would professionally encounter each other outside of it. Each differs varyingly from his "partner" in his expertise, educational background and professional code. Each has a traditional way of operating and a unique language. Attempts by these parties to operate together are further complicated by strong self-interest currents. To be effective in this kind of system, an individual player should have an appreciation of his "partner's" field. In actual practice, however, he may discover that areas of commonality are smaller than expected. A physician and attorney working together, for instance, are frustrated to learn that they cannot speak each other's language and that a discussion of the origins of a medical condition leads to ideas which seem to be incompatible. A human resources manager has an unreceptive audience when trying to convince a personnel officer that a certain supervisor is harassing his staff and causing many to file stress claims. He is dismayed to learn that the alleged perpetrator is more valued by the company and no remedial action will be taken. A claims adjuster insisting the treating psychiatrist file detailed progress reports is unaware of the critical role of confidentiality. Similarly, a legislator trying to improve the system's efficiency is criticized by the medical field when it never occurred to him that a conflict of interest dilemma is created when the treating professional also acts as the evaluator. Many other incompatibility problems surface among compensation professionals. All may block communication, undermine trust and jeopardize a cooperative effort.

Often a major compensation player doesn't know he is involved in a multi-discipline system. Accustomed to operating independently, he initiates a helping strategy without realizing he has precluded the contribution of fellow players. Only later does he discover that he cannot carry out his plan without "third parties," or even "fourth parties," and that recovery was prolonged by these unilateral actions. Adding to the complexity of a multi-party scheme is the human element—the individual operating style of the doctors, attorneys and examiners who make the everyday decisions about injured workers. The proper subject of the compensation professional is always an individual, someone not too different from himself, and arguably needed is a capacity to look beyond case loads, money issues or the medical-legal procedure. The operation of a compensation system is greatly facilitated by a willingness to ease self-interest, along with a deliberate effort to surmount the common emotions affecting the system, such as fear and greed. Benefits cannot be delivered smoothly in a multi-party system, and it is expected to have an adversarial quality.

The complexities increase at the clinical level as attempts are made to evaluate, treat or rehabilitate the injured worker. When any of the parties initiates action, fellow players feel they must do something to reassess or reestablish their own positions. If the worker's attorney obtains a psychiatric evaluation, the insurance company also requests one. If the doctor extends his patient's period of disability, the defense attorney suggests that the claimant's medical condition is not compensable. These actions, whether necessary or not, detract from the system's task of helping the worker recuperate from his injuries. Healing is delayed, disability prolonged and the patient placed at a greater risk for having psychiatric complications. Adversary activities increase the number of variables affecting the case and *prolong the time* the recovering worker remains in the system. Obviously, the longer the worker is exposed to the hazards of the system, the more complex his case becomes. With time alone, the negative reinforcers tend to gain momentum and impede recovery. The analogy of a pawn involved in a lengthy chess match has been drawn by many workers caught up in this industrial scenario.

The original condition for which the worker sought

treatment is overshadowed by a growing sense of frustration as he encounters these difficulties. Listening to workers describe this experience creates an impression that *relief from the mental strain of being in the system* is a more pressing issue than receiving treatment for the work injury. As he searches for both kinds of relief, the worker may discover that not one professional involved in his case has a comprehensive understanding of his needs or is in a position to do something about them. In a health care system where the need for a case manager is so compelling, there is no such provision.

In other health care fields, the role of case manager is traditionally played by the general practitioner. Internists and other specialists have moved into this area of medicine. This medical "agent" is a specialist in his own right. More than any other physician, he views his patient as a whole person and assesses his overall medical needs. His job is to personally direct the flow of his case to assure that assessment and treatment are performed properly and when his patient needs them. The closest thing to a primary care physician in the industrial system is the orthopedic surgeon, often the first specialist called to the emergency room to treat a seriously injured worker. The orthopedist, however, is not in a position to additionally serve as his patient's case manager. His interest in the musculoskeletal system is well-focused. Typically, he organizes his work day to maximize use of his special expertise, and the patient may not feel invited to tell his story. The doctor may not necessarily have an interest in his patient's total welfare or feel obligated to explore medical issues outside of his field. In a treatment delivery system which is inefficient and prone to psychiatric complications, the orthopedist may overlook the fact that psychological factors have entered into the clinical picture and are impeding his patient's recovery. He may be unaware that he is dealing with complicated forces about which he has little appreciation or formal training. In the simplest instance, the orthopedist may not realize that from the very beginning, his back case was a somatoform pain disorder superimposed on a minor sprain. In a system which is highly litigated, he may feel obligated to keep his focus narrow.

The chances are slim that the surgeon will refer his injured patient to a general practitioner or internist for purposes of overall management. Since there is no provision for payment, the worker may have to resort to a primary care physician outside the industrial system. Many workers lack the resources to enjoy such services or even health insurance. By virtue of entering the system by means of a physical injury, the worker is short-circuited from making contact with a generalist or internist, the professionals best qualified to assure timely evaluation and treatment. Others in the system who may appreciate the overall medical needs of the injured worker are his attorney or the claims examiner. But a legal agent cannot do the job as well as a medical agent, and a claims representative, however sensitive to the worker's problems, is primarily a case manager for his employer. Neither has formal medical training. Like the claims person, the occupational physician is hampered by conflict of interest pressures.

An example of a problem stemming from the absence of a qualified case manager is the lack of an accurate diagnosis. Without specific knowledge of pathology, treatment will be misguided. The forces shaping a worker's course of recovery are sometimes overlooked for years. In a compensation system, the number of these influences can be staggering. Somatoform disorders, the gains from disability, compensation grudges, a failure to grieve and negative bias may drastically reshape the course of recovery. Unless the industrial professional has intimate knowledge of these forces, the diagnosis will be missed. A common industrial scenario related to this is the absurd situation in which decisions are made about people who have non-existent medical conditions such as "post-traumatic syndrome" or "functional overlay."

The absence of a qualified medical agent leads to the more obvious problem of an inaccessibility to timely and appropriate treatment. A failure to refer to the proper specialist leads to a multitude of treatment pitfalls such as too much medication and repetitive monthly visits which are essentially useless. Too often proper treatment is not authorized when the patient needs it. The lack of timeliness may have real traumatizing effects. For instance, treating many conditions is only effective if rendered within a short time of the injury. These treatment "windows" may close early and never reopen. Phobic aversions associated with post-traumatic stress disorder must be addressed even more quickly. Treatment delays for most psychiatric conditions will result in chronicity or incomplete resolution. If the delay extends to a year or more, treatment could be for an entirely different condition. For example, if an adjustment disorder with depressive features is not resolved quickly, it may progress to a major depression or become complicated by panic attacks and agoraphobia. More commonly, untreated depressions lead to substance abuse and suicidal behavior. Among the compensation professionals, the qualified medical manager is in the best position to direct diagnostic and treatment activities. Even so, the worker may not be fortunate enough to be treated by a physician who appreciates the special influences and hazards of the system.

As a critically influencing factor, the industrial system may create a series of disasters for the recovering worker. The system's operation is slowed or paralyzed by its complexities. An inadequate diagnosis, improper treatment and delayed treatment send recovery on a downhill course. The length of time the worker is exposed to the hazards of the system is prolonged. The worker's condition becomes intractable, and he experiences excessive frustration. All of these complexities and shortcomings place him at risk for suffering psychiatric complications. The most destructive influence is that the system may contribute to psychological and physical damage which greatly exceeds that of the original injury. Chapter Four on the subject of the worker's psychological reactions to his injury will elaborate on these hazards. This chapter will also integrate material contained in Chapter Two about the nonindustrial elements and show how individuals with certain personality traits are expected to do poorly in a compensation system.

CHAPTER FOUR

The Grief Process and Injury

When a person is physically or psychologically injured, the injury becomes the central issue in his life and remains so until he recovers. During this time, the insult to mind or body will disturb his psychological equilibrium, and feelings such as depression, anxiety or frustration will be experienced to varying degrees. The industrial professional dealing with the worker expects him to be upset. But often he encounters such a bewildering commixture of emotionality and bodily distress that he might assume these responses defy explanation or analysis. The professional may not fully appreciate that the jumble of human distress before him reflects several overlapping psychological responses to the injury which are entirely predictable.

As outlined in Chapter One, a major injury, in terms of losing something valuable, is potentially the most psychologically traumatizing event of a person's life. An industrial injury may result in more than loss of a limb, a loss of a strong back or a loss of feelings of well being. There are equally devastating material losses such as a career, an adequate income, life goals, financial credit, personal possessions, or even his home or family. The worker is at risk for losing his self-respect, his self-image as a strong and effective person and his confidence for returning to work after a prolonged absence. During his recovery, a worker's problem-solving ability may be temporarily impaired. To make matters worse as he moves through the industrial system, decisions about his welfare will be made by others, and he may lose control of his destiny. All of these factors tend to reinforce each other and create a vicious circle of mounting personal losses.

Like the death of a loved one or losing a desired job, the losses associated with a major injury lead to predictable emotional reactions. The normal response to loss is a grief reaction. This is a circumscribed period of mourning which permits an individual to make the mental adaptation to his losses. Four predictable and well-defined stages in the grieving process can be identified—denial, anger, depression and resolution. Successful grieving will enable the worker to accept his losses and achieve a new psychological equilibrium. Following a major injury, the denial phase is very short, lasting only a few hours or perhaps lingering for a day or two. The worker who loses a limb, for example, may react with disbelief and refuse to look at his wound or communicate about his injury. It is too painful at first to face the harsh reality that he will be different forever and that he will have to undergo long periods of treatment and rehabilitation that will disrupt his life.

Denial quickly gives way to anger, as feelings of shock and resentment, concealed at first, come to the surface, and the injured worked tries to blame everyone, even fate, for his accident. At first, it is easier to lash out than feel the agony of a major loss. He is irritable with his family and resents his employer's inquiries about his health. He may change doctors or feel like filing a lawsuit at once. This phase usually lasts a few weeks. After this time, the intensity of his rage subsides, and the injured worker gradually allows himself to perceive the full impact of the lost limb on his being. Anger is followed by a sadness which pervades his life and evolves into depression. During this phase certain changes are noticeable to everyone dealing with him. There is a disruption of his eating and sleeping habits, moodiness, tearfulness and a tendency to draw away from everyone. He ignores his favorite activities and becomes preoccupied with himself. He communicates little and seldom ventures into the outside world. This phase may persist for many months. During the depressive phase the worker is preparing himself to continue life without the intactness of his body which he had enjoyed up to this point and which served him well in his occupational and personal life.

The stage of resolution begins when the worker anticipates the possibility that he may acquire new skills which will enable him to again operate as a viable and useful person. His sense of despair is replaced by an attitude of hopefulness, and he is more enthusiastic about participating in his physical therapy or his retraining program. The grieving process is nearing completion. As depressive symptoms fade, those around him observe a renewed interest in previous activities and friends, and daily activities become normalized.

Grieving has enabled the worker to restore his mental equilibrium. In this psychological process, a person builds an inner psychic structure which is different from the old one. This is a reorganization of mental life which takes into account the permanent alterations of his body and the changed circumstances of his life. Mourning is a normal human response to loss. Successful passage through this process is necessary if the worker is to accomplish the critical tasks of adapting to his injuries and resuming a productive and gratifying life.

Not all persons who have suffered a serious injury react in a psychologically normal manner. Sometimes the grieving process is sidestepped altogether. The losses associated with a major injury are never accepted. Even years after the accident, such individuals still struggle with the pain and shock triggered by this event. Permanent distortions in their psychological equilibrium result and condemn these persons to an unhappy and constricted existence. A more common abnormal psychological response to an injury is an incomplete passage through the phases of the grief reaction. A worker may become stranded in one or more of these stages.

This problem can be illustrated by my experiences with Denise, a never-married electronic parts inspector who suffered an amputation injury to about half of her right index finger in a machinery accident. She was referred for evaluation by her attorney because she was still unemployed two years after the injury and was making no effort to rehabilitate herself. Following the accident, Denise had developed an aversion for working around machinery, and her need to acquire new marketable skills had been recognized. But her aversion did not appear to be the problem. During the interview, Denise emerged as a very attractive, vain young woman whose dress and grooming were immaculate. She wore gloves but refused to allow me to see her injured hand. However, she ungloved her left hand to show me how the damaged hand had looked prior to the injury, going into great detail about the pleasure she derived from having long fingers and carefully shaped and painted fingernails.

At this time Denise told me a bizarre-sounding story of her search to find a healer who could restore her injured finger to its normal appearance. She was quite surprised when her treating surgeon informed her that the finger would not grow back, and Denise had spent a considerable amount of her own money to locate a surgeon who would attempt to reconstruct her finger. Denise also believed that regeneration was a distinct possibility, and she was convinced that ointments or potions existed which would stimulate regrowth. I got the impression she had already been exploited by a variety of pseudoscience practitioners. Denise told me about dreams in which she saw herself with a normal finger with a perfect fingernail like the rest. Her wish to have a restored finger consumed her life. When not seeking out healers, Denise stayed at home by herself. She refused to allow anyone to see her finger, including her immediate family, and she rarely permitted herself to view it.

It was evident to me that Denise had suffered a trauma to her self-image which had failed to heal. Vanity compelled her to hold tightly to the accustomed way of looking at herself not only as a physically attractive woman, but one who was perfect in all respects. Denise could not face the reality that the loss of her finger was permanent. Her energies and money were consumed by attempts to live in fantasy world in which this loss was temporary. From the examination I could see that the mutilating injury threatened to overwhelm Denise's precarious psychic equilibrium which, since childhood, was built upon a concept of herself as a physically ideal female. The emotional pain and shock from the accident was still present but held just below the surface by massive denial. Denise was consumed by a desperate attempt to keep her distorted and fragile equilibrium from further deteriorating. These preoccupations diverted her from the normal task of mourning her loss. It was clear to me that Denise had become fixated in the *denial stage* of grieving. Intensive psychiatric treatment, and perhaps a period of hospitalization, would be needed to help Denise overcome her denial and move through the grief process in the direction of acceptance of her injury. Until she had made considerable progress toward reaching this goal, attempts to retrain her would be futile.

A common problem encountered by workers' compensation professionals is a worker who has failed to pass through the angry stage of the grief process. This patient forever battles everyone involved in his case. All efforts to assist him in the recovery process are resisted. When plans are laid, he sabotages them. Attempts to communicate with him result in angry confrontations. As in Denise's case, the energies of such individuals are perpetually drained by intense emotion, in this case *rage,* whose purpose is to hold someone else responsible for the shock and bewilderment triggered by the accident. For some people, rage is a more tolerable emotion to endure than the emotional pain and shock of a major setback. To justify this intense anger, the worker desperately scans the external world for an explanation. Providing he can remain furious at his doctors, the insurance carrier, his employer or even fate, the worker can avoid experiencing the full impact of the injury upon his life. This is *an abnormal angry response* to his injury. The worker's anger pervades his life and fails to subside. This is different from the normal angry response to loss which disappears after a few weeks and evolves to sadness and depression.

It is the nature of the abnormal angry response to injury to feed upon itself and become self-sustaining. As the enraged worker searches the external world for somebody or something to blame, he invariably finds imperfection which is used to justify his angry responses. Following an injury, anger is perpetuated daily by reminders that he is a damaged person. His activity routine is impeded by a multitude of inconveniences and constraints. A worker with a deranged back, for instance, may be unable to perform simple repairs on his car or tend his garden. Overdoing it leads to many days of bed rest. He resents being deprived of pleasure-giving activities such as fishing or playing tennis. A person whose life has revolved around working can be enveloped in rage which is rekindled every morning when he cannot get up and drive to work as he has done all of his life.

Having to endure severe pain every moment causes a worker to have anger-induced preoccupations about being a victim of his employer's carelessness or greed. Or he asks endless questions about why he has become an accident victim, questions which have no answer and which serve to sustain his furiousness. He forever has thoughts about being "cast aside" inhumanely by his employer after many years of loyal service. Friends and family members who can work and carry on a normal life trigger *envy,* which like other painful emotion, is transformed into rage. Or a worker resents being supported by his spouse who was forced to work to make ends meet. Anger is fueled by the sudden appearance of many authority figures in his life. He blames his dilemma on the doctors, the claims adjusters or other practitioners in the industrial system. Every attempt to transact something with the worker is met with hostility which increases with each encounter.

The individual may remain suspended in the angry phase of grieving by directing this rage toward himself. He irrationally holds himself responsible for the accident. Thinking is dominated by ideas such as, "The accident wouldn't have happened if I had done that," or "I know I did something to deserve this."

Energies are consumed by endless reconstructions of the accident as he searches for evidence of his carelessness. This self-blame should not be construed as a willingness to accept responsibility for his dilemma, as it is merely another way to indulge in activities which impede normal grieving.

Regardless of its focus, rage takes over the worker's life and excludes other kinds of emotion or points of view. Like Denise who was locked in denial, the worker reacting with abnormal anger has failed to make an adequate psychological adjustment to his injury. Both suffer from genuine psychiatric illnesses which constrict their occupational and social lives. Clinically, this maladaptation may lead to symptom formation which meets the criteria for a psychiatric disorder. When the abnormal anger response to injury contributes strongly to physical symptoms such as pain or immobility, a somatoform pain disorder or conversion disorder may be diagnosed. Abnormal anger interferes with the administration of proper medical care and greatly hinders the work of rehabilitation.

Still other workers fail to effect passage through the depressive phase. Normal grieving is stalled by a deep sadness which pervades the worker's life for years. This common industrial condition is not to be confused with the normal depression of mourning, a temporary state of sadness which follows a major personal loss. The *abnormal depressive response* is far more severe and pervasive. It produces characteristic physical and mental changes and interferes in all areas of a person's functioning. Without treatment, it deepens and leads to profound unhappiness and disability. Such individuals never see any prospects for a future. The mood of depression is painful, and most of its victims have recurring wishes to die.

The unbearable nature of this pain was dramatized by the behavior of depressed patients I treated in Vietnam. They often communicated a willingness to trade the pain of their depression for the physical pain of men in the surgical tents nearby who had suffered loss of limb injuries and other combat wounds. My patients felt hopelessly trapped in time and space. They could not remember having significant past lives or envision futures for themselves. Such individuals experienced their lives as compressed into a single moment in the present, a narrow time frame which was unending and unbearable. They looked to the relief afforded by suicide, or they tried to numb pain by not caring about anything. These men felt alienated from other people. They isolated themselves for days in the tent wards and were oblivious to events taking place in the outside world. They manifested exactly the same changes I later observed in industrial cases when severe depression occurred as a complication of a physical injury.

For example, the illness of depression disrupts normal eating, sleeping and activity patterns. A depressed person feels slowed down in body and mind. He has little energy or endurance. Sometimes he is agitated and restless. Thinking and speech are slowed. Mental clouding is very common. A depressed person may be unable to organize his thoughts, remember significant events or focus his attention long enough to read or follow conversations. Thinking through and solving day-to-day problems may be difficult. Working or handling domestic responsibilities may be impossible. Feelings of self-confidence and self-worth are lowered. Such persons experience inappropriate guilt and reproach themselves. Like my angry patients, they were tormented by feelings of envy. As their depressions deepened, they felt increasingly inferior to and less worthy than others.

One of the prominent features of the abnormal depressive response is a tendency for its victims to experience aches and pains in virtually every part of their bodies. My patients in Vietnam reported on migratory bodily pain, but these symptoms posed no diagnostic or treatment problems. In the industrial system, however, soreness on a psychogenic basis creates many medical-legal dilemmas. A worker with a low back syndrome or cervical strain may have a component of musculoskeletal distress which is *caused by depression.* In this common industrial scenario, a worker's intense emotional reactions cause soreness, spasm and restricted movement which is *superimposed* upon the soreness and stiffness produced by the original injury. This makes assessment of the physical component bewildering. The task is complicated by the tendency for depression to alter a person's threshold for perceiving pain. In this response to injury, mind and body react together and converge on the musculoskeletal system, the site of the original industrial injury. The occurrence of proliferating aches and pains following a physical trauma suggests that the patient is reacting to the injury with severe depression.

Differentiating between physical and mentally-induced pain is perhaps the most difficult challenge faced by industrial practitioners. This clinical phenomena is commonly associated with treatment failure and delayed healing.

Workers with a primary psychiatric injury, such as a post-traumatic stress disorder, also react with their bodies and minds to the injury. Evidently, there is an area of our psyches which monitors the *intactness of our minds* as well as the intactness of our bodies. When mental functioning is disordered, humans will react with the same kind of denial, anger and depression outlined earlier in this chapter. In this respect, the patient with a stress disorder is no different from someone who has lost the use of an arm. Both must make a psychological adaptation to a health loss which is altering their lives. In this scheme, a worker who is unable to cope with a post-traumatic stress disorder may react abnormally by developing a separate and distinct psychiatric condition such as agoraphobia or alcoholism. This illness is superimposed on the original injury. It is entirely analogous to the depression which arises secondarily to a low back problem. Even a worker with a major depression may react to his illness by feeling even more depressed. It is not too difficult to see how psychiatric injuries become self-perpetuating as a worker's emotional reactions to his illness become mutually reinforcing.

Psychiatric injuries are also accompanied by losses, and they must be mourned as well. A person with a stress disorder may be so withdrawn that he loses his capacity to relate normally to coworkers or his family. A corporate manager with a major depression is plagued by self-doubt and indecisiveness which results in the loss of his ability to lead and a demotion. Similarly, an individual with a panic disorder can lose his ability to move freely within his environment. The denial, anger and sadness accompanying normal grieving are also set in motion by suffering these psychologically-related losses.

The fact that we can react intensely to the loss of our mental health is illustrated by my experiences with Norma, a married mother who found a job with an electronic manufacturing company after her children entered school. Norma had a college degree and a keen sense for business management. She moved up quickly in her company and within five years was promoted to a middle level manager. Able to thrive on long hours and heavy responsibility, Norma enjoyed her job. She was a perfectionistic, goal-oriented person who knew how to motivate people and get results. Her undoing occurred when the company had a slow sales year and laid off many workers to cut losses. Because of her excellent track record as a manager, Norma was retained. In the consolidation process, however, Norma was given the managerial responsibilities ordinarily handled by several people. While everyone had to work harder, Norma's duties increased the most. Her supervisor voiced confidence in her, and Norma poured her energies into her job. However, the load was too heavy, even for an energetic person like Norma, and within eight months she collapsed at her desk from physical and mental exhaustion.

Following her collapse, Norma couldn't stop crying or screaming at family members. She was unable to get a full night's sleep and had no desire or stamina to do anything. For days at a time, she stayed in the house, refusing to answer phone calls and leaving domestic chores to her husband. Her most distressing symptoms were crying spells and an inability to use her mind normally. She couldn't read or follow conversations. Four months of psychiatric treatment and being away from the demands of her job failed to have a beneficial effect on Norma's condition. She resented her employer's calls about her condition and wrote vitriolic letters to the claims adjuster.

Referral for psychiatric evaluation was made by the industrial carrier when it appeared that Norma's mental status was deteriorating.

During the evaluation, Norma emerged as a proud woman who had high standards of occupational performance and personal behavior. As I listened to Norma talk about her job, I could not escape noticing her perfectionistic traits and workaholic approach to life. Moderate depression was also present. Norma was a far cry from the robust and healthy person suggested by her history. She was quite aware of the drastic changes in her mental health, and her self-image as a strong and competent person had eroded away. I was convinced that Norma's reactions to her illness were entirely normal. All of her life she had enjoyed a being a strong, invincible and psychologically stable person. Prior to this illness, nothing had occurred in Norma's life to challenge this image. It was evident that Norma was reacting intensely to the loss of intactness of her psychological well-being. She had never been emotionally out of control before. Her energy was always boundless, and she never suffered from fears or doubts. Being unable to think normally was an entirely new experience.

From the evaluation, I obtained strong evidence that Norma was going through the normal process of grieving the loss of her emotional stability. An initial period of *denial* was evident from the history. Symptoms of exhaustion, emotional lability and mental clouding had preceded her collapse by three months. She ignored them and carried on as if nothing were wrong. Norma secreted her distress from her supervisor and her husband. Prior to her illness, Norma hadn't slept for a week. She covered up this fact by claiming she was up late in their home office to do "reports." At work, Norma ran almost hourly to the restroom to hide her tears. In the emergency room Norma demanded that the doctor return her to her job at once. Denial quickly gave way to *anger* when her personal physician placed her on medical leave and her employer insisted that she have a period of rest or treatment.

During the next few weeks, Norma was livid. She resented her employer's calls about her welfare, and she screamed at her husband. Having to come for the interview was infuriating. But during our discussion, I saw that Norma's angry feelings were rapidly fading away and that she was feeling quite depressed. Norma spent much of the interview telling me how her "breakdown" was incomprehensible to her. To shore up her self-image as a strong person, she talked at length about her past achievements, frequently interjecting remarks such as, "I was always a confident, strong person," or "This is devastating to me," and "Why couldn't I do that job?"

As we talked, it became clear that after a period of denial and anger, Norma was permitting herself to face the painful reality that she had suffered a serious psychological injury which would have lasting effects. Sad feelings and a willingness to perceive all of her psychological reactions to the illness were reliable signs of a healthy involvement in grieving. While Norma could not step back into her previous assignment, I felt she had an excellent prognosis for returning to a managerial job with less responsibility. She had good basic psychological strengths and was devoted to working. Norma's emotional reactions to her "breakdown" were normal, and I was able to assure those involved in her case that with time and treatment, she would do very well.

The final phase of the normal grief process is *resolution.* In this phase, the injured worker must consolidate the gains made in the three previous stages and find a realistic way to resume a productive and gratifying life. In psychiatric terms, the goal of this stage is closure—the crucial move of putting the traumatic episode behind and stepping into a new life. During resolution, the worker is expected to encounter certain obstacles. Following a long period of recuperation, feelings of confidence for returning to a competitive work market will sag to some extent. It is entirely normal for the person in this situation to worry about the quality of his up-coming performance.

During resolution, the reappearance of problems thought to have been resolved is exceedingly common. A low back syndrome may flare up or depressive symptoms may suddenly return. This is a normal and expected psychological reaction to being released for work, and is not to be construed as a recurrence of the original condition.

In the final phase of grieving, the worker must come to grips with the financial losses associated with his injury. A worker in the construction trades, for instance, will have to accept the harsh reality that the sedentary occupation he is entering offers a lower income. An office worker may not earn as much as a plumber or crane operator. The stage of resolution is the time for a "final accounting" of gains and losses. Before accepting a closure of his case, a worker must face the likelihood that overall, his injury has resulted in a net loss. He must accept that the industrial system does not compensate the worker for all of his losses, and there is no provision for the inconveniences and suffering forced upon him by the accident.

Another normal adjustment required of a physically-oriented worker during this phase is coping with *mental stress* at work for the first time in his life. While a construction worker may have endured physical stress for years, he may be surprised to discover that an office worker feels an entirely different kind of pressure. It is normal for workers who are on the eve of returning to their jobs to worry about a reinjury. A temporary aversion for the occupation hazard is expected.

During resolution, a worker may deal with any of the above obstacles in a psychologically abnormal way. Long beyond the time his injury has stabilized, self-doubt about his abilities may grow and keep a person away from the work place. A worker's loss of confidence may be so profound that the expected flare-up of his symptoms during rehabilitation may persist, and compensation professionals will find themselves back to "square one." The final accounting of his losses may stir up feelings which are too painful for the worker to bear. To avoid them, he will sabotage his training program or find other ways to postpone settlement. A blue-collar employee may not be able to make the adjustment to white-collar work and forever become fixated in this late stage of grieving. During this critical time, excessive concerns about reinjury may balloon into full-fledged phobic aversion. The risk for this complication is especially high if the offending hazard has not been corrected. I have not encountered an injured worker who has failed to find out through the grapevine whether or not the faulty machinery, for instance, has been repaired before returning to his job. In Norma's case, complete grieving and a return to the work place would not be expected unless she received assurances, ahead of time, that her work load would be more reasonable.

In addition to a normal grieving, it is useful for industrial professionals to realize that workers respond psychologically to their injuries in other normal and predictable ways. Serious injury to a bodily system is an emergency condition to human beings. To maximize survival of the organism, a person's physiologic resources are temporarily concentrated upon the damaged system. While these energies are thus redirected, the functioning of other systems will be impaired. A major injury will normally compromise a person's ability to cope with demands and pressures from the outside world. Problems which he usually handled with ease may be experienced as overwhelming. In this situation, a person can be expected to undergo some degree of psychological regression. Helpless and childlike behavior become noticeable. His way of solving problems becomes more ineffective, and he may be unable to protect himself from further adversity. For these reasons, the recovering worker has a *heightened susceptibility* to additional insult or injury.

This increased vulnerability has an adverse effect on the course of the worker's original injury as he moves through the industrial system where he must contend with additional stressors. As pointed out in Chapter Three, the system tends to let the worker down when his needs are the most pressing. As these negative factors come to bear upon his welfare, there is a growing danger that the worker's psychological responses to his injury will be abnormal. Ensuing feelings of frustration, anxiety, anger and depression feed upon themselves. Depression causes him to ache all over, and psychic disequilibrium interferes with his ability to deal with pain. At this point in recovery, a patient loses his ability to distinguish between physical and emotional pain. Long after the injury has healed, the worker continues to believe he has physical derangement. The worker is further bewildered by his doctor's insistence that nothing is wrong with him.

When a worker is physically or psychologically injured, he becomes more vulnerable to the stressors impinging upon him from every area of his life, including the industrial system. He is more susceptible to further injury, and he will remain so until he recovers. He becomes psychologically regressed, and his ability to cope with demands or pressures is reduced. Minor annoyances are experienced as being overwhelming, and major problems become traumatic events. While recovering, he is more emotionally unstable than before, and his psychological symptoms tend to increase before they improve. The seemingly confusing emotional reactions of injured workers can be understood in terms of these normal and abnormal responses, both to his original injury and to the stressors he encounters as he participates in the industrial health care system.

For the reasons outlined, there is a high incidence of abnormal psychological responses to all types of industrial injuries. In turn, these abnormal reactions place the worker at increased risk for developing psychiatric complications. They also increase his chances for experiencing delayed healing, unexpected disability and treatment failure.

CHAPTER FIVE

Secondary Gain

Doctors and nurses are always distressed by the fact that not all of their patients want to get well. It is a true paradox than anyone would prefer illness over health, or disability over being fully functional. Yet, the motives of such a patient can be discovered if certain practical gains from the illness or injury are considered. It is understood that sick people are privileged in industrial societies, and a worker with a severe malady knows he can be excused from his job. But when there are compelling reasons to be excused, and no malady exists, one will have to be invented. This happens commonly in the industrial system when an employee enhances the effects of an accident to stay home. In this scenario, the desired result is referred to as secondary gain. Its name is based on the assumption that what is gained is derived secondarily from the symptom or disability. In the thinking of the worker, the benefits he seeks would not otherwise be obtainable. The secondary gain might be something obvious such as avoiding an angry boss or more subtle such as disguising a personal inadequacy. In each case, the symptoms are of paramount importance to the individual and will not be easily relinquished. For this reason, secondary gain issues are a *total obstacle* to the treatment and rehabilitation of the injured worker.

Obvious as this kind of human phenomenon might be, defining it precisely is difficult. Is secondary gain a psychiatric condition, a behavioral maneuver, a mental aberration or perhaps a psychological ploy? The texts in psychiatry and occupational medicine appreciate the role played by secondary gains in these fields, but the topic is never discussed at length. Seldom is more than a paragraph devoted to it, and the contents are limited to a suggestion that the reader already knows about the gains from illness, and there is a reminder of its importance. More information about secondary gain is found in the psychoanalytic literature, but impreciseness of terms often obscures it meaning. Analyzing the obvious is difficult, and writing about it is tedious. The search for a practical definition of secondary gain is complicated by a need to explain its role in two other conditions of interest to compensation professionals, malingering and the somatoform disorders.

Two examples of somatoform conditions—conversion disorder and somatoform pain disorder—are often encountered in a compensation system, but they are apparently rare in the private sector of psychiatry. They evidently exist because strong secondary gain forces are at work. Even a layman understands that the malingerer has certain gains in mind, and that a patient with psychogenic paralysis of his legs, for example, is desperately struggling with a personal problem. This raises the additional question: Is secondary gain the cause of a psychiatric condition? Before attempting a definition of secondary gain which is workable in an industrial system, its role in malingering and somatoform disorders must first be described.

Malingering is defined in DSM-III-R as "intentional production of false or grossly exaggerated physical or psychological symptoms, motivated by external incentives such as avoiding military service, evading criminal prosecution, obtaining drugs, or securing better living conditions." Intentional means that the individual experiences a sense of having control over his symptoms. Here, the motive of the malingerer in terms of receiving benefits is identical to that of a worker who is enhancing his injury to be off work.

In the case of somatoform disorders, the same concept about motives holds, as DSM-III-R describes their essential feature as "physical symptoms suggesting physical disorder (hence, Somatoform) for which there are no demonstrable organic findings or known physiological mechanisms, and for which there is positive evidence, or a strong presumption, that the symptoms are linked to psychological factors or conflicts. Unlike malingering, the symptom production in Somatoform Disorders is not intentional, i.e., the person does not experience the sense of controlling the production of the symptoms." It is now clear that the motives of a worker with conversion disorder are the same as the malingerer since he is altering certain aspects of his bodily functions to cope with problems and obtain personal advantages. The essential difference at this point is a matter of conscious control.

A definition must also account for the widespread use of the term "secondary gain" to account for the origins of conversion disorder and a psychogenic pain disorder. Anyone who is curious about these conditions learns that two psychological mechanisms explain their appearance. In one, *primary gain,* the person keeps a personal conflict from his awareness by *converting* a mental disturbance to a physical one. DSM-III-R describes the other, *secondary gain,* as follows: "In the other mechanism, the person achieves 'secondary gain' by avoiding a particular activity that is noxious to him or her and getting support from the environment that otherwise might not be forthcoming."

This is awkward, as it sounds like secondary gain is being offered as the origin of these conditions. Something is missing, and this seems to be a convenient way to describe the mental activity which leads to the achievement of secondary gains. The concept is clarified if a term such as "secondary gain mental mechanism" is used. This phrase suggests that the mind is taking action to cope with a psychological disturbance by first converting it to a bodily symptom, and then using the symptom to get something from the external world. If this manipulation works, there will be some resolution of the psychic dilemma. Redundant as it may sound, the worker employs a "secondary gain mental mechanism" to obtain secondary gains. This mental *maneuver* can be viewed as the origin of all somatoform symptoms. While little is known of the neurophysiological processes taking place in the mind when this mechanism is activated, the result is a complex, and sometimes successful, form of problem-solving behavior. This term is very useful since it provides a way to refer to the *psychic activity* which brought about the end result or "secondary gain."

In a compensation system, "secondary gain mental mechanisms" can be used to describe the origins of a wide variety of somatoform symptoms. For instance, it may be identified as the cause of chronic back pain when there are no physical findings. It explains the clinical phenomena referred to as "functional overlay." This is an expression used by nonpsychiatric physicians to record their impressions that psychological factors are influencing the patient's bodily complaints. Another term—"secondary gain behavior"—can be used to accurately describe the *observable actions* taken by the worker as he implements his plan. Similarly, an expression like "secondary gain issues" has practical value since it can serve as a convenient way to address this subject in a general way. For instance, "secondary gain issues" can be discussed by lawyers and adjusters with the same facility as they discuss treatment issues or disability issues in a case. When communicating about this subject from an even broader viewpoint, the term "secondary gain phenomena" used earlier in the chapter can take on a precise meaning.

From this, it can be seen that the malingerer, the

patient with a conversion disorder and the worker who enhances his disability to stay home, are all doing the same thing. All are taking action to resolve a psychological dilemma by converting it into a bodily symptom, and then using the complaint to obtain something from the external environment. This psychological scheme is fairly complicated, and a single definition falls short. Secondary gain has various facets, and additional terms are required.

To begin with, *secondary gain* is the objective attained from a certain kind of mental activity and behavior. The psychological activity in this scheme is a *secondary gain mental mechanism,* and the observable actions taken by the worker to achieve his aim is *secondary gain behavior.* When this kind of activity is discovered in a compensation case, it becomes *a secondary gain issue.* The subject as a whole can be referred to as *secondary gain phenomena.* For the remainder of the chapter, these terms will be used as this subject is developed in detail. The essential ingredients of secondary gain phenomena will become even more clear as case illustrations are offered.

Clinically, secondary gain behavior may be *unconscious* or *intentional,* and this may have an important bearing on the medical-legal aspects of the case. One or the other may be evident to an industrial manager. On close study, however, varying elements of each may be encountered in a given case. For example, a secretary may not realize she is enhancing the effects of a minor injury to be off for two weeks. But this can be acknowledged when her husband points out that her department is currently being relocated, and that she wants to spare herself the frustrations of the move. He reminds her of the debilitating headaches she had the last time the office was moved and the secretaries were expected to carry boxes and the computer equipment.

Secondary gain phenomena are universal, and they probably have been in existence as long as mankind. Our ancestors who benefitted from miracle cures over the centuries were probably individuals who activated secondary gain mental mechanisms to avoid working, not unlike some of their modern counterparts. The clinical acumen of their healers must have been excellent, considering that in reversing a case of paralysis or blindness, they could identify secondary gain behavior and determine which symptoms were organic and which were psychogenic. There is nothing exotic or mysterious about these phenomena. They are an inherent part of everyday life, as most of us can recall at one time or another having invented a minor malady to excuse us from an unwanted situation. The motive is universally recognized. Hollywood writers often use secondary gain behavior as a comical device in motion pictures and sitcoms.

A memorable example is the scene in *Charlie and the Chocolate Factory*, in which Charlie's grandfather, Papa Joe, overcomes a longstanding debility. In the movie, Charlie holds a ticket to Willie Wonka's famous factory, but as a condition of admission he must be accompanied by an adult. Seizing the opportunity at once, Papa Joe, bedridden for years, miraculously arises and dances a jig with Charlie. His grandfather can relinquish the care afforded to a physical invalid when there is far more to be gained as a guest of the fabled Willie Wonka. A secondary gain mental mechanism may be applied to any human dilemma which calls for a quick and desperate remedy. It may be activated to resolve an old psychological conflict. Or it may be used to fulfill a long-frustrated need. As so often happens, secondary gain behavior may be inspired by a chance event.

The opportunity may be an industrial accident. Nowhere else is the occurrence of secondary gain phenomena so prevalent as in the arena of industrial accidents. The occurrence of an injury provides a person with a special status. He is doubly privileged by the attention afforded to injured people and the practical benefits owed to him by his employer. He is in a position to take advantage of these considerations by prolonging recovery or intensifying his symptoms. This special status tempts a worker to attribute medical or psychological problems irrationally to industrial events which may be trivial or non-existent. There are many ways to resolve a personal problem, and using an unrelated illness for this purpose is not very effective. Presumably, the workers who try to solve problems in this manner have limited resources for coping with difficult life situations and personal frustrations. Considering the high price they pay in terms of pain, disability, financial loss or constriction of their lives, the situations from which they seek relief must contain elements which are even more miserable.

Since the purpose of these mental maneuvers is to enjoy certain personal benefits, the worker will not give up his symptoms easily. He holds them as a ransom to get what he wants. Remaining sick is a *guarantee,* and treatment and rehabilitation are unwanted. The medical records of these patients usually reveal a *paradoxical response* to treatment—they get worse rather than better. Traction or a corset, for instance which might be expected to afford partial relief of back pain, causes discomfort to increase. These individuals develop unusual complications to diagnostic procedures, and surgical results are often disastrous. The therapist senses the disabling symptom is a valuable possession which is clutched more tightly as he tries to eliminate it. Secondary gain behavior such as this will totally defeat the efforts of compensation professionals to return these individuals to work. These issues must be clarified and worked through if treatment and retraining are to be effective.

The kinds of personal advantages to be derived by this are nearly endless, as there is no apparent limit to the variety of problems which beset human beings. Money is probably not the most common secondary gain encountered in the industrial system, although it is the most obvious one. Most secondary issues arise from problems in relationships. Disruption of the family system is a very common trigger. It can be recalled from Chapter One that Ross exaggerated his neurological symptoms following a head injury in a desperate attempt to get his family back. While this maneuver failed, Ross had not yet developed other means to deal with his painful loss. A worker may also prolong his symptoms to win back an estranged lover, a rejecting parent or a child who is about to establish independence. Getting back in good standing with a group of friends or coworkers after being disgraced or falling out of favor may also be accomplished by exaggerating an injury.

An example of *successful* secondary gain behavior of this kind occurred in Vietnam where I was assigned to the psychiatric department of an Air Force hospital. Each morning, hundreds of Vietnamese civilians entered the sprawling base at Cam Rahn Bay to fill jobs in its operation and perform houskeeping chores. The women were highly social and worked together in closely-knit groups of twenty or more. Every few weeks, an ambulance would be dispatched to pick up a "seriously or fatally injured" Vietnamese on the base premises. The scene of the accident was predictable—a lone figure, seemingly unconscious on the ground, surrounded by a growing hoard of panic-stricken or crying coworkers. Examination of the patient, however, revealed only a minor bruise or scratch, and sometimes no apparent injury. Making the diagnosis of psychogenic unconsciousness was not difficult. The injured was loaded onto the ambulance, and the group of coworkers jogged behind, continuing to express their anguish in the most dramatic ways imaginable. Our patient received first aid for her wounds if necessary and was placed in a quiet area of the tent-hospital. In the meantime, coworkers kept an agonizing vigil outside. All work was halted. In an hour or two, our patient emerged spontaneously from her "coma." When their injured companion was escorted out of the hospital intact and apparently healthy except for a few bandages, the mood of the group changed from despair to joy, which was expressed personally to the patient in an equally vociferous way.

Vietnamese interpreters provided a history of the "accident" which was as predictable and uniform as the clinical picture. The incident was usually something minor like tripping and falling, or the result of a scuffle. Before this event, however, our patient had been castigated at length by the group for some offensive behavior and was in the process of being ostracized. The grave "injury" or even "death" of the companion whom they had just mistreated evoked sufficient guilt to stay this form of group punishment. In the "miraculous" recovery of our patient, the collective guilt of her coworkers was supplanted by a swell of joy. All was forgiven, and she was returned to the group as an honorable member. For our patients at Cam Rahn Bay, grossly exaggerating trivial injuries may have been the optimal solution to a desperate problem. In the setting of a bureaucratic and business-oriented society, however, this kind of manipulation is less effective, but it may serve a limited purpose for the worker.

Numerous other kinds of personal dilemmas may occur in *close occurrence* to an industrial accident. Like Ross, workers with such problems may exploit their injuries to solve them. Another illustration is the case of Armand, a truck dispatcher in his early fifties who developed unexplained pain in his knee after undergoing surgery for a torn ligament. He was referred for psychiatric examination because of depression. History revealed that after fifteen years of being single, he impulsively became engaged to a long-standing friend. The proposal took place after the accident, and it was mainly at his fiance's insistence that

Armand agreed to corrective surgery. The wedding was scheduled at time when full recovery from the knee operation was anticipated. Post-surgically, Armand did poorly. He complained of intractable pain and an inability to bear weight. Doctors were baffled by the surgical result. A secondary gain mental mechanism was identified. I sensed that Armand regretted his decision to remarry, but he was unable to perceive his true feelings and could not call the engagement off. However, with Armand physically immobilized, almost broke, and his life at a standstill, the wedding had to be postponed. His fiance was frantic and became involved in every aspect of his life, including his medical care. This attentiveness markedly aggravated his knee problem. Armand's depression deepened, and he overdosed on pain medication.

It was readily apparent during the evaluation of this unhappy person, that being a near-invalid served the useful purpose of avoiding an unwanted marriage. He accepted my referral to a therapist who encouraged the couple to talk about their true feelings. When this could be done, the engagement was mutually broken. Since Armand's pain and disability now served no purpose, they quickly cleared, and he returned to his dispatcher's job. Armand's poor response to surgery was a two-pronged psychological strategy, unintentional as it may have been, to sabotage his upcoming wedding. As a near-invalid, Armand could not be expected to honor his marriage commitment. At the same time, he could discredit and then devalue his fiance since it was her idea to submit to an operation that went poorly. While Armand's secondary gain mechanism eventually worked, he endured unnecessary hardships which almost destroyed his life. His experience is a good illustration of the unpredictable and inefficient nature of this problem-solving technique.

In addition to resolving a personal crisis like Armand's unwanted engagement, a disability may be magnified to deal with *current problems at* work. Examples include harassment, heavy work loads, hazardous job conditions or accountability pressures. Prolonging recovery may be the worker's only way to avoid these noxious job elements. Not all of us have the means to handle adversity well. There are many people who lack the self-assurance and assertiveness needed to complain about difficult work conditions. Overly afraid of being fired, they bottle up frustrations and endure in silence. An industrial accident is a welcome event, since it affords much-needed relief which they might not otherwise enjoy. These people are highly prone to secondary gain behavior after an injury. Treating and returning them to their jobs is frustrating. Some workers lack the capacity to recognize and express even ordinary negative emotion such as irritation or resentment. When dealing with a provocative boss or coworker, they cannot show reactive anger because they do not recognize it. Instead of voicing resentment as most people would do, these individuals get back at their employer by prolonging their symptoms. Staying sick to retaliate for past mistreatment may be referred to as a compensation grudge. This form of secondary gain behavior is common among anger-inhibited people.

Frequently, secondary gain mental mechanisms are activated *after an injury* when a worker encounters problems during recuperation. The circumstances which give rise to most of these problems are the frustrations of being involved in a multi-party compensation system. Not receiving a disability check on time or waiting for approval of treatment can stir up sufficient resentment to trigger a compensation grudge. Much of the delayed healing, treatment failure and unexpected disability encountered in industrial cases reflects an attempt by workers to retaliate for perceived mistreatment during recovery. These grudges are generated by other frustrations. Workers often experience a loss of control over their lives. They may lose their homes, automobiles, their credit rating, their paramours or family. Some frustrations are more subtle. For example, an injured worker often experiences the system as omnipotent and uncaring, and his own position as powerless. In this situation, remaining disabled is a means to influence his destiny. While this behavior may be destructive in the long run, the achieved gain of having some control over one's fate, meager as it is, may boost a worker's self-respect. This shred of power may be the only thing that sustains him during a prolonged and difficult rehabilitation.

A common secondary gain occurring during recovery is avoidance of a job environment in which management has failed to eliminate the hazard which contributed to an accident. A waitress in a busy restaurant had several trip and fall accidents from loose floor tiles on the ramp leading to the kitchen. Others had tripped on the same spot, but complaints were ignored. Eventually the waitress sustained a shoulder injury which led to an unexplained period of disability. As the sole provider for her family, she desperately needed the income from her job, and a secondary gain issue was identified. During the interview, she talked at length about her employer's cavalier attitude toward the unsafe conditions faced at work. The claimant told me she had returned to the restaurant to inspect the damaged floor area, but to her dismay no repairs had been made. There were even more loose tiles than before, and she began to keep count! While the waitress denied that the unrepaired floor could delay healing, I was convinced otherwise. It is easy for such an oversight to become a *symbol* of the neglect or mistreatment felt by the worker in connection with the accident. Feelings of hurt and anger are attached to the neglected hazard, and a compensation grudge may be created. For this worker, a repaired floor would be interpreted as a sign from her employer that he cared.

Similarly, victims of harassment usually remain symptomatic until steps are taken to protect them from the offending supervisor or coworker. Secondary gain behavior may be a way to cope with stressful changes taking place at work. For example, being reassigned to a supervisor the worker dislikes or having his department moved to an undesirable location may cause a worker to prolong his recovery. Yet another reason for enhancing symptoms during recovery is the forestallment of a termination which is expected when the doctor signs the release.

The changed circumstances of a person's life brought about by an injury may generate a secondary gain mental mechanism. The simplest example is a worker whose disability income exceeds or approximates his lost wages. When this happens, the incentive to work may vanish. Another example is a person who has worked steadily for 30 years or more. While recovering from an injury, he may decide that his work life has come to a natural end and he is ready to retire. This is seen mainly in laborers, whose careers began in childhood or early adolescence which is often the case among migrant field workers. Sometimes, a person in a highly stressful occupation experiences a sense of relief during an involuntary absence from work. As a result, he questions his interest in returning to it. Similarly, a person in a highly skilled or competitive field may lose his confidence for performing adequately after a long absence.

In these examples, workers experience a forced interlude from their occupations which are then viewed from a different perspective. The achieved gain is an honorable release from duties which they no longer want to perform or believe they can perform.

An illustration of this behavior was a warehouse manager in his early sixties who sustained a fractured neck vertebrae when he was struck by a falling stack of pallets. In six months, his neck condition had stabilized.

When he returned to his old job, debilitating neck pain appeared unexpectedly, and he was never again productive. The manager was not required to perform physical work, and there was no apparent reason why he could not be a supervisor as usual. A somatoform pain disorder was diagnosed. A secondary gain mental mechanism was readily apparent during the evaluation. Upon returning to the warehouse, it was evident to the younger workers that their superior had suffered a loss of his powers of command and authority. They no longer respected him and were frequently insubordinate. The manager told me they played cruel tricks on him such as hiding his lunch pail or tacking up caricatures of him on the bulletin board. Disabling neck pain enabled the manager to spare himself this humiliation. At the same he could disguise his inadequacy and retire for a respectable reason.

Sometimes an injured worker prolongs recovery to obtain a grandiose cash settlement or unrealistic rehabilitation program. In this form of secondary gain behavior, symptoms are held in ransom in hopes of winning the desired benefit. For example, a mechanic with a deranged lumbar spine resisted getting well so he could pursue admission to law school, a venture he expected his employer to finance. A factory worker who couldn't read extended recovery for years while he insisted the carrier help him open a business. In these cases, the worker is having difficulty accepting the painful reality that he will not be fully compensated for his injuries and will actually suffer a net loss. The desire for an inflated settlement is an attempt to deny this eventuality. Similarly, a worker may activate secondary gain mental mechanisms indefinitely because closure will cause him to face his losses and feel painful emotion. An additional form of secondary gain behavior during convalescence is the spontaneous appearance of a non-industrial health problem such as arthritis for which the worker would like to be awarded medical treatment.

Here, the worker extends the symptoms of his industrial injury so that they incorporate or blend with his non-industrial condition.

Workers also prolong their disability in an attempt to solve problems which have been in existence *long before* their industrial injury. During my treatment of Marion, a 40 year old accountant with multiple injuries, I encountered a secondary gain issue which concerned a family problem troubling her for more than 15 years. Marion was struck by a table which had been propped up behind a storeroom door, and she developed severe shoulder and hip problems. Doctors could not explain her failure to heal and made a diagnosis of a conversion disorder. Psychiatric treatment was recommended because she was severely depressed. Two years after the injury, Marion still lived at home as a near-invalid. She was very proud of her family ties and always got along well with her husband, teenage children and family of origin in which she was one of twelve children. Her husband was college educated and made a good income. They had done far better than any of her brothers and sisters. While Marion and her husband were buying a large home in an affluent neighborhood, her siblings were floundering.

Eventually, Marion's denial about having family problems broke down, and she told me the following story. Ever since her marriage, Marion's relatives had freeloaded on them shamelessly. An endless parade of siblings brought their children and spouses to Marion's home where they lived for a period of time, eating their food, wearing their clothes and using their cars. At a given time there were about six extra people in the home. Sometimes her children had to sleep on the floor. Marion catered to them without question or complaint. This role was instilled in her since childhood. Her elderly parents often called to remind Marion that her brothers and sisters couldn't get by without her. Marion's husband handled the situation by having affairs and avoiding the home as much as possible. In therapy, the rage and frustration connected with her desperate family situation slowly surfaced, and Marion began to say no to her relatives. She also reestablished her relationship with her husband. As a final solution they moved to a distant state, and Marion recovered sufficiently to find a job. Marion's near-invalidism was a desperate plea for relief. She was helpless to deal with her family problems directly since her role as the family caretaker seemed natural and normal. It was not until this secondary gain mental mechanism was clarified in psychotherapy that Marion learned the real origin of her physical and emotional problems.

A poor work record is commonly encountered among workers who present with intractable disability. It is important to take a careful work history and to ask specific questions about the annual incomes of such workers. For example, I learned from a totally disabled office worker with a master's degree that the most he had earned in a year was about five thousand dollars. The hoped-for gain from his illness was a reliable source of income. Some workers have felt insignificant all of their lives and have always held menial, low paying jobs. The event of an industrial injury provides them with an opportunity to feel *important.* A worker with an intractable and unexplained disability receives much attention from doctors, lawyers, judges and other compensation professionals. Being the focus of special concern for a prolonged period is evidently worth the price these individuals pay in terms of being debilitated.

Similarly, many people go through life feeling disfranchised, that is, without a place to belong or without power or privileges. They feel like they are on the outside of society looking in. An industrial disability may afford them some *entitlement.* Feeling as if they own something overshadows any material benefits which they might derive from the injury. A person with a long-standing dependency conflict may respond to an industrial injury by acting totally helpless. In these cases, the secondary gain of being taken care of by others exceeds the wish to have an adequate income.

Because secondary gain behavior blocks the efforts to return workers to their jobs, it must be identified and eliminated. Understanding the complicated interplay of personal and industrial factors which gives rise to these phenomena is one of the most difficult tasks of the industrial professional. Early recognition of psychiatric disorders is so important to effective management that Chapter Nine will be devoted to this subject. In order to maintain the continuity of this subject, early recognition of secondary gain issues in a case will follow in this chapter.

■ ■ ■

The search for a secondary gain mental mechanism begins by building a familiarity with the worker in the entire context of his life—past and present and anticipated. This includes learning about his age, culture of origin, childhood experiences, family configuration, religious beliefs, enduring personality traits, occupational history, important relationships, successes and failures, his past methods for dealing with adversity and a medical history. Leads can be developed from the narrative history, medical records, personnel file or from information provided by friends, coworkers and relatives. Look for a person who can benefit from a disability—someone who has been struggling with a frustrated wish, an unfulfilled need, a desperate crisis or any other human dilemma. Think in terms of a "sticky" or "sensitive" problem, one which places the worker in an unflattering light. Always be on the alert for a person who has poor problem-solving techniques or limited work skills.

Identifying secondary gain issues early-on requires an

aggressive approach. The patient cannot always be expected to know about his problems, as the workers who utilize this primitive way to cope with problems tend to have limited powers of introspection. For this reason, compensation professionals must inquire about areas of a worker's life which are claimed to be conflict-free. Early recognition depends upon a strategy of identifying *potential* problems, those which are not apparent on the surface but which can be inferred from the available information. When approaching stress injuries, it is helpful to use the analogy of piecing together a jigsaw puzzle. Many of the pieces can be connected easily, but some take a long time to find. Those already in place suggest the appearance of the missing pieces. In industrial cases, trying to construct the missing area of the picture is as critical as studying what can be seen.

After becoming familiar with the worker, an industrial professional can focus more intensely on aspects of a worker's life in which there are potential problems. For example, a person who recently moved from a rural community to a more cosmopolitan one may be unable to adapt to the greater pressures and faster pace of the city. An anger-inhibited person may not be aware of an intimidating situation at work or home, and it would be necessary to inquire in detail how he gets along with supervisors, coworkers, his spouse and the other important people in his life. A working mother may have a husband who has enough income to support the family on one pay check, and she may not be motivated to work. Someone in his late 20's or early 30's who is still living at home may be prolonging his disability to counter parental pressure for him to move out and establish independence.

Early recognition of secondary gain issues depends upon having a high index of suspicion of all cases in which *healing is delayed.* This subject will be elaborated upon in Chapter Nine but is introduced here as it applies to recognizing secondary gain mental mechanisms. Compensation professionals must realize as quickly as possible that an injury is responding poorly or having a downhill course. Unexplained pain, unexpected loss of function, a paradoxical response to treatment are some of the early clues that secondary gain mechanisms are at work. Further clues are the spontaneous appearance of new complaints, the extension of symptoms to other areas or involvement of multiple bodily systems. Look for physical symptoms which are commonly caused by emotional distress such as headaches, sore muscles, stomach distress, dizziness, faintness, feelings of weakness, tiredness or an appetite disturbance.

The medical records provide the earliest clues of all. They contain information that the injury was relatively minor or trivial and that inconsistencies and discrepancies were already noticed by coworkers or physicians. The records may reveal an attitude of puzzlement or suspicion by the first group of treating doctors or consultants on the case. Later the records may state that objective signs of injury cannot be found. They reveal multiple diagnoses, no diagnosis or a pseudodiagnosis such as "functional overlay" or "chronic fasciitis." Other valuable clues are the prescribing of much medication, numerous consultations and changing modes of treatment. The presence of these elements in a case is a clue that an injured worker's course is not going as expected and that the doctors are frustrated.

Evidence of a potential or existing psychological problem in an injured worker's life, combined with an unexplained disability, suggests that a secondary gain mental mechanism is influencing recovery. The benefits obtained from his symptoms are highly valuable, and until relinquished will defeat the efforts of compensation professionals to treat and rehabilitate him. The predictable results are the complications seen in industrial injuries, such as treatment failure, delayed recovery, unexpected disability and psychological invalidism.

CHAPTER SIX

Why Treatment Doesn't Work

The conditions under which treatment takes place have a critical bearing on the outcome of a stress injury. For psychiatric treatment to be effective, certain time-tested ingredients must come together. Unfortunately, the industrial health care system creates settings which are not conducive to a good result. To begin with, confidentiality by legal mandate is not preserved. With perhaps several doctors, two lawyers, a claims representative, a rehabilitation counselor, a state agent and a judge involved in a case, it is difficult to imagine how therapy of a mental disorder could work. Complete privacy is ordinarily required to encourage an individual to share the most sensitive and intimate aspects of his being, and without this, psychotherapy is often useless. In a compensation system, treatment takes place in what might be described as a crowded fishbowl. This setting might be expected to promote distrust and inhibit communication of emotional material. What the patient tells the therapist is colored by the fact that his comments will influence decisions made by third parties about his job, disability income or settlement.

Another example of unsuitable treatment conditions is a lack of timely diagnosis and therapy. Initiation of treatment is related less to the needs of the worker than to the plodding and seemingly capricious nature of the multiparty benefit delivery system. By the time therapy is authorized, treatment windows may have closed, and chronicity already set in. Treatment may come so late that it is for a different condition. For example, a harassed worker placed on a leave because of anxiety and shakiness may end up with a major depression and a substance abuse problem if treatment is postponed. Delays permit secondary gain issues such as a compensation grudge to invade the clinical picture and undermine treatment.

Distractions impede the treatment of a psychiatrically injured worker. With normal income interrupted, setbacks occur in his personal life. The worker may be forced to change his residence, lose his automobile or suffer disturbances in family relations. The energies of therapy are drained by these distressing events. It is difficult, for example, for a therapist to treat a disabling depression when his patient has been evicted from his apartment and abandoned by his girlfriend. Litigation pressures ordinarily shove treatment issues to the side. Unresolved questions about the eligibility of a claim result in treatment which is fragmented or contaminated by distrust.

Or worse, these activities place treatment on hold or disrupt it altogether halfway through. Even when therapy is authorized, legitimate needs to monitor it are distracting to both patient and therapist. The spontaneity of the treatment process is blunted by having to tell the same story over and over again to outside evaluators and testers. The psychotherapist is inhibited when there are legal pressures to break confidentiality and furnish information to third or fourth parties. In a compensation system it is practically impossible to keep privacy and skirt conflict of interest problems. Even when an effort is made to minimize them, the conditions of treatment may not be adequate for a good result.

Compared to other health care systems, the industrial sector does an ineffectual job preparing an individual for psychiatric treatment. Much training is offered to therapists about the importance of readiness for using psychotherapy, and the resident psychiatrist learns that half the work of therapy takes place before his patient comes to the first session. Optimal conditions for treatment are illustrated by the private pay (or private insurance) patient who is aware of good reasons for seeking help. He is very worried about himself and determined to make good use of psychotherapy. He comes because he wants to, and he is willing to share in the responsibility for getting well.

The private patient is self-referred, or he finds his way to the psychiatrist or psychologist through his primary care physician. A clergyman or other professional helper familiar with the benefits of psychotherapy may make the referral. More commonly, he is encouraged to call the psychiatrist by family members or a network of friends and colleagues. Often these individuals have been in therapy themselves and can provide useful information about using this treatment. Ahead of time, the private pay patient has some idea that he will have to work hard to derive any benefit. Treatment is properly looked upon as an investment in his time and money, and he must use it efficiently. There are practical considerations, as he must find a resolution to his difficulties before his money runs out.

The industrial patient bears little resemblance to his counterpart in the private pay sector. He comes to therapy late in the course of his dilemma, and he may already have a chronic condition. The industrial parties in his case missed the diagnosis for months or years, or they ignored it or passed the buck. Unlike the general physician or clergyman, a compensation professional may not regard psychiatric referrals to be part of his professional role. Even if willing, he may lack the training or expertise needed to prepare his patient for therapy. More technically-oriented physicians feel uncomfortable about confronting emotional material. Perhaps the commonest reason for failing to refer is a busy style of operating which allows no time to get to know the patient as an individual.

Very often, there is a reluctance to uncover what may be a new injury or claim.

Too often when the psychiatrically injured worker comes, he is a reluctant patient. He tells the psychiatrist that the referral was someone else's idea and doesn't understand what can be done to help. His visit is perfunctory, and he doesn't expect to continue. No one has taken the time needed to win his trust and discuss the reasons for referral. Further reducing his chances for success, no one prepared him for a facilitative approach in which the therapist is not expected to do all the work. Patients who don't know this beforehand misperceive psychotherapy as another remedy offered by medical science in which their role is merely that of a passive beneficiary. For instance, this was the expectation of a city worker in his forties who was convinced the psychotherapist could quickly remedy his lack of self-confidence and tendency to invite the badgering behavior of coworkers. Without an appreciation for the true nature of therapy—a facilitative or enabling process in which the patient assumes the responsibility for changing himself—such persons may become disillusioned and drop out after a session or two.

Workers with pervasive child-like or adolescent traits are evidently at high risk for having a stress injury, and many find their way into the industrial health care system. They have always lacked the self-assuredness to direct their own lives, and not unexpectedly, they want industrial professionals to solve their problems. Curiously, they interpret the obligations of the compensation system literally: those who have "deprived" them of their health have a duty to "cure" them. This attitude is incompatible with an effective treatment, since therapists lack "curative" powers and psychiatric treatment is fundamentally a shared undertaking. These unrealistic attitudes pose a stiff challenge to the psychotherapist. When injured, these workers shift the responsibility for getting well to others. They become helpless and demanding, and many are not candidates for psychiatric treatment in the first place.

Because they lack resources to fall back upon, many undereducated and disfranchised persons depend heavily upon the industrial health care system. Conventional treatment seldom works with these injured workers. They lack sophistication about mental and bodily functions and tend to experience anxiety and other forms of mental anguish in the form of *physical pain.* When they suffer back or limb trauma, intense fearfulness causes them to perceive the injury in a greatly magnified way. Unless this emotional component is identified, their failure to respond to treatment can be truly baffling. Special treatment conditions are required, such as referral to someone who understands somatization problems, or treatment by a therapist who is attuned to their culture and can react with sensitivity to their lack of knowledge or superstitions. Educational and cultural considerations aside, many people are not able to perceive emotional reactions or even to appreciate that they have inner lives. Unless a special set of treatment conditions is offered, these individuals will be unable to use outside assistance to recover from their physical or emotional injuries.

Whether or not a patient is working plays a critical role in therapy. In nonindustrial cases, the patient is not ordinarily disabled. He is actively involved in the outside world, and brings into therapy sessions his conflicts precisely as they occur in the arena of his day-to-day life. A problem he had at work on Monday is discussed with the therapist on Tuesday. This lends to a favorable outcome. The sessions are "live," enabling the psychotherapist to clarify his patient's difficulties in the context of here-and-now situations. A disabled worker has no such advantage. His problems occurred in the past, and in therapy they seem abstract or intangible. The sessions have a "dead" feel, and the only here-and-now issues are how boring it is to stay at home watching television or waiting for something to happen in his compensation case. Treatment cannot take place in this kind of "vacuum." To benefit, the worker must be actively involved in the very areas of his life where he is having problems.

For instance, someone who finds himself disliked by coworkers cannot sharpen his interpersonal skills unless there is an opportunity to test himself in "live" situations such as the work place. Often doctors are overly eager to place symptomatic patients on a medical leave. While this enables them to feel quick relief, it dilutes the potency of psychotherapy as a way to resolve human dilemmas. When the absence from the work place is lengthy, the risks for treatment failure are increased. A better strategy is to encourage the patient to return to his job and face his problems. Any subsequent failure to resolve them can be brought into the sessions and serve as the psychological medium from which more effective behavior can grow. Even when a disability leave is unavoidable, an early return to work is a useful subject to talk about in the next few sessions. Years of clinical experience have convinced me that a get-well-first-and-return-to-work-later strategy simply doesn't work.

Even when the above problems are avoided, treatment conditions for an industrial case may still be unfavorable. Optimally, the worker has a therapist who understands the unique influences of a compensation system. He is familiar with the natural history of industrial accidents—that a myriad of unique forces will endanger his patient's welfare—and he is skilled at keeping recovery on track. Ideally, the psychotherapist has a knack for recognizing obstacles posed by secondary gain behavior and those which are culturally determined. He is skilled at facilitating the grieving process, while helping his patient sidestep the pitfalls of the system. He understands his patient's vulnerabilities and is flexible enough in therapy to do whatever is necessary to speed his patient's return to work. Above all, the effective industrial therapist realizes that he and his patient are running a race against time, and that the longer his patient must depend upon the industrial system, the worse his prognosis will be. A therapist with these qualifications is not always easy to find.

There is a greater chance that the worker with a stress injury will be referred to someone who is fairly inexperienced with industrial accidents. The system by nature is self-contained, and not many practitioners appreciate its scope or its ways. The peculiar aspects of compensation injuries are usually ignored in formal training programs, and a therapist can labor for years with a stress case before acknowledging that unaccountable forces are at work. In the simplest instance, treatment fails because the psychotherapist doesn't see that secondary gain issues have entered the case on a delayed basis. Unconsciously the patient places more value on his disability than he does in being fully functional.

The principles of psychiatric treatment and what a psychotherapist does to conduct his work are beyond the topic of this book, but certain fundamental tasks can be sketched out. Choosing the proper treatment is one. Traditionally, therapists are trained to have a thorough understanding of mental disorders, and familiarity with a wide variety of treatment modalities. After a comprehensive assessment, the therapist must select the treatment which works best with a certain condition. Psychoses, for instance, may be approached best with hospitalization and medication in the beginning stages, with a change to a supportive type of psychotherapy and maintenance medication following a remission.

Severely depressed patients are frequently candidates for mood elevators, and lithium maintenance is ordinarily a mainstay for bipolar disorders. Adjustment disorders may quickly remit with brief psychotherapy and a few weeks of medication. Individual psychotherapy has proved to be the most effective treatment in a wide range of personality disorders and neuroses as well as for post-traumatic stress disorder. Group therapy is more effective in certain types of disorders such as chemical dependency.

A "talking therapy" may be selected, and as treatment proceeds, the task is to keep a constant eye on the patient's inner world. The therapist learns of his strengths and weaknesses, his fears, moods, hopes and frustrations. Familiarity is gained of the individual in the context of his past life, and of his repetitive way of dealing with others and coping with adversity. Note is made of how he is dealing with current forces in his environment.

Gradually an understanding of his patient's mental life comes, and the psychotherapist faces the next task which is to create a dynamic formulation of his case. A formulation is an explanation of the patient's psychological life and behavior, and it contains a summary of the forces which gave rise to the illness. Dynamic, as opposed to static, means that the patient's behavior is constantly being influenced by certain forces whether they are psychological or environmental. The patient generally reacts predictably when encountering these forces. The inner or psychological determinants of behavior are often referred to as "the psychodynamics" and are relied upon heavily to conduct therapy. The formulation acts as a stable guide for what is often a complicated and occasionally bewildering undertaking. Ordinarily, this road map for treatment changes very little, and most experienced therapists don't bother to write it down (although written formulations are a major training tool during residency training.) Another task in this simplified description is setting the goals of therapy.

These goals are mutually agreed upon and must be appropriate to the diagnosis and the overall life circumstances of the patient. They may be short-range such as resolving a crisis, or ambitious such as making a major change in the person's way of operating. Realistic objectives lend stability and clarity to the therapeutic process. In addition, they enable progress to be accurately assessed. Preserving confidentiality is a critical task, and there is an agreement to keep outside distractions to a minimum. By the time these basic chores are underway, the therapist is applying time-tested ways to facilitate change or resolution of conflicts. There are other dimensions common to all forms of psychotherapy, such as resistance, regression and transference, but in the limited scope of this chapter no attempt will be made to describe them. Instead, the focus will be on how difficult it is to accomplish even the most fundamental tasks of psychotherapy in a compensation system.

While making an initial diagnosis is seldom a problem, the patient's mental state may change drastically and unexpectedly as he encounters the industrial health care system. As described earlier, its pitfalls can have real traumatizing effects. The following case is an illustration of these difficulties. A roofer in his twenties is diagnosed as having a post-traumatic stress disorder after a life-threatening fall which damaged his legs. He suffers from nightmares, anxiety, insomnia, irritability and headaches. He is withdrawn and avoids his friends and family. The fall caused him to have a phobic aversion for being in high places, even above the ground floor of buildings. Treating him will not be easy.

While disabled, he will be expected to face one crisis after another. The accident is the worst thing that ever happened to him, and he lacks the psychological maturation to deal with it constructively. In addition to a stress disorder, the therapist finds his patient to be an adolescent-like individual who is easily frustrated and who has a history of reacting with anxiety and depression when under stress. Within a short time, the patient falls into a severe depression. A talking therapy along with mood elevators to relieve depression is the chosen treatment regime. But medication makes the young man feel worse, and he falls into a deeper mood state. Antidepressants must be abandoned, and it is difficult to know what to focus on in therapy. At this point it is not clear if the depression is an aspect of normal grieving or a delayed or unmasked depression from the fall. Considering the young man's personality disorder, the therapist must assess the risk that his depression may become self-perpetuating if disability is prolonged, and that grieving (if in fact it is the depression of grieving) will never be completed.

Psychotherapy enables the young man to talk about the impact of the accident on his life, but this is interrupted when he faces his first setbacks. His disability checks are not sent on time, and therapy is put on hold while he is sent to psychologists and psychiatrists for evaluation. His employer then calls and communicates annoyance because of the expenses and inconvenience caused him by the injury. The worker's reactive anger to his boss's telephone call markedly increases his other symptoms. For weeks, the treating doctor encounters nothing but paranoid-sounding ruminations about his employer. Now the therapist's job is even more complicated. He doesn't know if he is treating one, two or even three superimposed conditions, and making a formulation is bewildering.

Confidentiality has long been violated, and the numerous distractions are washing over the structure of therapy and breaking it down. Upsetting events are happening almost on a weekly basis, and the patient cannot keep all of his appointments. It is nearly impossible to accurately assess the patient's mind. The therapist has an impression he is trying to zero in on a moving target.

Slowly, the system responds to the worker's medical and rehabilitation needs, and the young man begins to feel a little better. There is less anxiety and depression, and his nightmares are subsiding. He contacts his old friends and finds a new girlfriend. His fear of heights diminishes and no longer constricts his movements. However, the role of therapy in his improvement is uncertain. The therapist still doesn't have a stable or reliable formulation. The process is repeated as the worker faces other financial crises and personal losses. The young man requires surgery on his legs, and recovery is prolonged for more than a year. His patient reacts with marked helplessness. The problems for the therapist continue, as he isn't sure whether to interpret this behavior as the normal regression which accompanies a major injury, an aggravation of his character disorder or an early sign of chronic invalidism. The therapist decides that a secondary gain issue is now stalling progress. The young man's frustration and rage are not subsiding, and he is unconsciously staying disabled to express retaliation, not only against the parties involved but against fate for causing the accident.

An additional setback occurs when the worker learns that he cannot return to construction work. Again he falls into a severe depression. While this depressive reaction seems to represent normal (and healthy) grieving over the loss of his career, the psychotherapist is little comforted. The forces impacting man's recovery on an almost weekly basis preclude the luxury of having a reliable guide for assessment and treatment.

At this point, it can be seen that even the task of setting therapeutic objectives is frustrated by the set of treatment conditions faced by the worker and therapist. While alleviation of depression is a presumed goal, it is too ambitious because of the numerous reinforcers encountered during recovery. Facilitating a healthier psychological adjustment to the leg injury is difficult because of his deeply-rooted maladaptive character style. Providing emotional support during recovery is a risky objective since it might increase helpless and dependent behavior. Even normal grieving is difficult to promote since the numerous developments in the case would make assessment of this process impossible. Because of mounting losses and insults during recovery, the worker's post-traumatic stress disorder and personality disorder are repeatedly being aggravated. Even though the patient is not yet recovered from his physical injury and still emotionally unstable, a question can be raised about continuing treatment. Few in the way of tangible benefits have been provided, and a lengthy treatment would probably delay the initiation of self-reliant behavior.

Since treatment conditions are far from optimal, the therapist and patient probably have done as well as they could. The problems they faced are common in a compensation system. When a physical injury is complicated by a major depression, there is little the psychiatrist can do since the worker's mood disorder will usually have a course parallel to his pain and disability. The psychotherapy of an industrial stress injury is a much larger and more complex task than treating nonindustrial disorders. Considering the high incidence of secondary gain behavior, maladaptive character styles, a need to grieve losses, the hazards of the system and suboptimal treatment conditions, it is not surprising that the psychiatric treatment of an industrial stress injury often doesn't work.

Much research into the treatment of industrial conditions is needed. It has already been suggested that flexible or unconventional approaches work better. A greater appreciation for diagnosing and treating Axis II conditions is needed. Similarly, anyone who treats industrial injuries must be familiar with cultures and socioeconomic stations which are different from his own.

CHAPTER SEVEN

Negative Bias

A compensation professional makes decisions about an array of business, financial and medical-legal matters, but his essential concern is an individual who has a problem. Managers have to be good psychologists. It can be shown that university presidents, football coaches, or corporate managers who are preeminent in their field have a profound knowledge of human behavior and of how it can be influenced or directed. A professional who is sensitive to people and able to view an injured worker as someone not too different from himself will have an advantage over someone who lacks curiosity about human behavior and who experiences a troubled person as strange or alien. A major handicap such a manager might have in this regard is a *negative bias* about workers who claim psychiatric problems. The main influence of this attitude is that it leads to decisions about injuries based on emotion, misinformation or traditional prejudice rather than objective information. There may be many different reasons for this inclination.

A professional encountering a worker who has a psychiatric disorder may confront intense human emotion such as frustration, rage, despondency, terror and suicidal wishes. He is faced with demands to be taken care of and urges to get back at someone. He will constantly have to contend with manipulative behavior. For months or even years, he will assume some responsibility for a person whose life has come to a standstill and who is floundering in many areas of functioning. The industrial practitioner discovers that his efforts to help are misunderstood, and he finds himself the target of misdirected hostility. As a result, he may feel infuriated and drained. These workers can stir up in the professional the same out-of-control feelings. Dealing with such claimants can make him feel close to losing his own control, his cool or his professional objectivity. For all these reasons, his responses to these persons can be negative.

At the same time, the behavior of these patients may be truly baffling. Yet none of us likes to find ourselves at a complete loss for understanding. Admitting ignorance is unpleasant, and most of us prefer to display our expertise. In this situation, it is typical of human behavior to invent an explanation. While involved in discussions about stress cases, I have heard contemptuous remarks like, "Anyone knows psychiatric problems are easy to fake," and "He belongs in a psychiatric environment, not in my office" and "Those people just have poor protoplasm." More than once I was confronted with, "If a worker chooses to feel that way, it's his problem." Everyone in the compensation industry has encountered ideas about psychiatric disorders similar to these. But such an "explanation" of human behavior misses the mark so widely that it is not a genuine attempt at understanding but a *tacil denial* that psychiatric disorders exist at all. In this kind of thinking what is not understood doesn't exist, and what is encountered before our eyes must be attributed comfortably to something familiar as determined by misconceptions, a lack of intimate experience or slanted attitudes.

From these comments, it is clear that workers who claim stress injuries can be viewed by industrial professionals as having something wrong with them which is outside of the medical field. Allegations of psychiatric illness can be dismissed on the presumption that anyone who deviates so noticeably from ordinary human behavior must be an alien, a complainer, an incompetent, a goldbrick, a laggard, a shirker or a scoundrel. This point of view is only a short distance from the conviction that workers claiming stress injuries are evil, contemptuous, amoral, substandard or deficient in some other way. This thinking has not evolved very far from an explanation of mental illness popular several hundred years ago which held that psychotic people were witches controlled by the Devil. Such distorted notions still exist in our society (Casella, 1986), and mental illness is deemed by many as a mark of disgrace. Persons looked upon this way will be treated with reproach. Because of these widespread attitudes, there is a high risk that workers who claim disabling stress problems will become the "lepers" of the compensation delivery system and will be avoided.

My first experience with the potentially destructive influence of negative bias occurred during my tour of Vietnam where I was assigned to an Air Force psychiatric hospital at Cam Rahn Bay. A group of airmen was hospitalized with a severe adjustment disorder immediately upon arriving in Vietnam. They were reacting to the unpleasant prospect of a 12-month tour of duty in a primitive jungle environment. Like the rest of us, these men had to endure constant heat, humidity, filth, vermin and dangers. Added to these were psychological stress elements such as delay, shortages, uncertainty and ambiguity—factors which crept into everything a person tried to accomplish. Most of us endured in the face of hardship and futility, but our distressed patients became dysfunctional and looked forward to a medical evacuation. Often they were brought to the hospital hyperventilating, crying and unable to walk. Comrades reacted to these pitifully-acting men with disdain and rejection. Unit commanders did not want them back, and higher-placed military officials were willing to oblige. Usually, they were labelled as "complainers" or "misfits." It was expected that they would be flown to a state-side hospital and administratively separated from the Air Force. Prior to the opening of the Cam Rahn Bay hospital in early 1966, this had been the typical disposition of these airmen.

However, when they were examined closely from a psychiatric viewpoint, ways were found to treat them in-country and in all cases return them to their original units. None were psychotic, and their histories suggested they were anything but misfits. There was a disproportionate number of career servicemen in this group, and all had a good prior military record. Prior to assignment to Vietnam, there was no indication they might have psychiatric difficulties. Our staff discovered that the eagerness to assign a pejorative label to these troops and be rid of them was motivated by their tendency to make commanders and fellow airmen feel uncomfortable. They were living reminders that, we too, were vulnerable to reacting badly to the miserable conditions of Vietnam. If honest with his feelings, hardly a person in Vietnam could deny wanting to regress or go home. But this was unmanly or unwomanly, something most of us trying to perform our duties would not like to know about, let alone admit.

In psychiatric terms our patients were suffering from separation panic. They had deeply-rooted dependent personalities which made them susceptible to emotional problems when assigned away from their spouses or family. Unable to adapt to this separation as most of us were trying to do, these men became unstable. It was not until they could be understood as persons with a special vulnerability—and not too different from the rest of us—that treatment could take place. While in the hospital, it was possible to alleviate panicky feelings by use of individual psychotherapy. A major step toward recovery was enabling them to see that separation from family was merely temporary. Returning these men to their units was facilitated by helping commanders regard them in a different light. In this group which consisted of 30 men, all completed their tour of duty in Vietnam.

In the industrial system, there is a similar viewpoint that something is wrong with you if you have a psychiatric problem. Decisions influenced by negative bias cause workers to be seen as misfits much like our patients in Vietnam. Such thinking may take on other forms. An employee who has a psychiatric disability may be regarded as having an improper attitude. He may be deemed as lacking in will power or good judgment. This worker would stop feeling miserable if he had more determination or a better approach. In this scheme, his unhappy predicament is no more than "just desserts" for being lazy or failing to use the right kind of thinking. A simple change in outlook would solve his problems and enable him to regain control of his life.

But human distress eludes simple explanation, and none of these ideas sheds meaningful light on psychiatric conditions. On a case-by-case basis the situation is quite complicated. Just because there are workers who have fraudulent personalities or maladaptive traits doesn't necessarily mean that a stress claim filed by this person is fraudulent (although it might be), and the fact that faked injuries *do* exist doesn't mean that *all* claims of psychiatric injury are simulated. There is no way to determine the legitimacy of a stress claim until the evidence is examined in depth.

Psychiatric claims are no different in this respect from alleged injuries to the lumbar spine, shoulder, heart or brain. For the reasons already developed, a preconceived notion that a worker's stress claim is fraudulent is a product of negative bias. It is possible, of course, to be right for the wrong reasons, and the worker in question may turn out to have a contrived injury after all. The idea that psychiatric symptoms are generated by forces beyond the interest of the medical field is absurd, as a person cannot turn a depression off and on like a faucet no matter how hard he tries.

It is useful to be skeptical in managing industrial claims, but the most important caveat is not to become jaded. No one would dispute the need for a high index of suspicion for malingering in a medical-legal system. But failing to remain equally alert for a genuine psychiatric disorder is an indication of negative bias. Detecting the malingerer in the compensation system is difficult, and this subject will be discussed extensively in the following chapter. This chapter will also describe how the weeding-out process greatly distracts from other management, treatment and rehabilitation activities.

Negative bias about psychiatric conditions is a critical determinant of the course of stress injuries since it places the industrial professional at high risk for losing objectivity. When this happens, decisions are made to increase his own comfort and have little to do with the merits of the case. The destructive effect on the worker with a genuine injury is that his case is neglected, and he is additionally traumatized by hostile attitudes. Accurate assessment is postponed indefinitely, and treatment comes too late. The critical influence of negative bias is that it contributes to prolonged recovery and unexpected disability. Sometimes, the trauma of such bias can lead to a separate psychiatric disorder which is superimposed on the original injury.

CHAPTER EIGHT

Pseudoindustrial Injuries and Malingering

Sometimes an adjuster must contend with the claim of an injury which he suspects has *no link* to the work place. This leads to a management dilemma. On the one hand, the examiner has an obligation to deny benefits to ineligible claimants, yet in making this determination, he doesn't want to create a hardship for workers who have compensable injuries. This is very difficult to do. Weeding out false claims is time-consuming, and it subjects a person to unfamiliar and stressful inquiries. While attention is focused on these activities, the task of rehabilitating the worker with a genuine work injury is suspended. Expensive as this weeding-out process might be, it can be even more costly when it is delayed or carried out inefficiently. The predictable extra costs to both worker and system are in terms of delayed treatment, prolonged recovery, excessive disability and psychiatric complications.

False claims take two forms which are differentiated by the element of conscious intent. The first are claims in which unconscious mental mechanisms compel a worker to blame a personal difficulty on something which happened at work. Because these conditions are falsely attributed to his job, they can be referred to as pseudoindustrial injuries. The second type of false claim concerns a disability which is deliberately produced and which fits the DSM-III-R definition of malingering. Timely recognition of these two conditions enables the examiner to keep the management of bonafide work injuries on track.

Pseudoindustrial injuries occur when a worker tries to disown a long-standing or recent personal dilemma by attributing it irrationally to his job. Here, the problem is severed from its origins and connected to an event at work which is then placed to the forefront. With the truth momentarily disguised by the claim against his employer, the individual can show his emotional distress without having to feel responsible for it. In a simple illustration, a worker rejected by a lover suffers a debilitating depression. To deflect this blow to his self-esteem, he attributes his painful mood state to a critical comment made by his manager. In a more complex case, a worker from a foreign country is unable to make enough money to sponsor the immigration of relatives. To ward off a sense of failure, he unfairly accuses his employer of holding him back because of cultural prejudice. Or, an individual who has never made more than poverty-level wages, attributes his poor mental health and dismal life situation to a trivial slip-and-fall accident. In each case, the worker absolves himself of any shortcoming and blames his employer.

Workers make false claims of injury because they are trying to shift the responsibility for a personal crisis to external factors. In the face of life's minor setbacks, this kind of behavior is apparently normal. Most of us blame others momentarily when things go wrong in our lives. If our income tax bill seems too high, we may believe our accountant is incompetent. When a paper error is called to our attention, we may accuse a coworker of supplying the wrong information. If our favorite football team loses an important game, few of us can resist blaming the officials. Admitting a personal failure, even a small one, may stir up transient feelings of embarrassment or inadequacy. It is natural at first to spare ourselves this painful emotion and point the finger elsewhere. We presume that workers who file these claims are facing dilemmas outside the work place which are far more serious and might be upsetting to almost anyone. The search for these problems is critical to an effective management of cases in which there is a question of eligibility.

Pseudoindustrial injuries are illustrated by the case of Vera, a 28-year-old woman who lived at home with her aunt. Vera's alleged back injury occurred two months into her employment as an aide in a convalescent hospital. One day, she noticed progressive soreness of her lower back and legs, and after getting off duty she drove herself to a nearby hospital. In the parking lot, Vera's legs became very weak, and she collapsed on the floor of the emergency room entrance. She was unable to move her legs, and the doctors admitted her for a comprehensive evaluation. Nothing physical was found to explain her "paralysis," and after a few days in the hospital, she could ambulate with a walker. Her mobility slowly increased, but weakness and bothersome leg pain persisted for months. By the time I evaluated Vera for a suspected conversion disorder, she had filed a claim of back injury against her employer and was living at home as a near-invalid.

Vera knew little about her parents except that both had died in an accident when she was an infant. She was raised by an aunt who divorced before Vera was eight years old. The aunt had never remarried and devoted her time to Vera. In the interview, she made no effort to disguise the fact her aunt did everything for her. Vera had never learned to cook, clean, make her bed or arrange her clothes. There was no expectation to do homework, and with her aunt's permission she dropped out of school during the tenth grade. Vera never dated. Her only friends were women her aunt's age. Twice, she had moved out to live with them; however, when expected to share expenses, she returned home where her aunt demanded nothing. The clinical examination was in keeping with the history, as Vera emerged as child-like person who was content to live at home and enjoy the indulgences of her aunt. What convinced me that Vera's leg symptoms had no connection to her job was the information offered that several weeks before the alleged injury, her aunt revealed plans to remarry. Vera was shocked. At the same time, relatives and friends were more outspoken about her moving out and becoming independent. She was especially upset when her older friends were unreceptive to the idea of her moving in with them. She did everything in her power to dissuade her aunt from marrying, even initiating some unflattering rumors about the fiance.

It was clear that Vera was facing a major life crisis related to the loss of her aunt as an indulgent parent and pressures to grow up and become self-sufficient. Her solution was immature and maladaptive. Becoming a near-invalid was a manipulative attempt to cancel her aunt's expectations for adult-level behavior. Vera's conversion disorder was entirely determined by this personal crisis. Claiming a job injury served the dual purpose of offering her aunt a reason to continue infantilizing her, and relieving Vera of any responsibility for her dilemma. Like Vera, many individuals use the industrial system as a repository for an insurmountable personal difficulty. The most useful way of discovering them is a systematic study of the worker in the entire context of his life.

Perhaps the most distracting element an industrial professional must deal with in managing a stress injury is the phenomenon of *malingering*. In this condition, there is a claim of symptoms or a disability which is intentionally produced to obtain obvious external incentives such as compensation benefits. As noted in Chapter Five, there are varying degrees of deliberately—and unconsciously—produced symptoms in a given case. For instance, it is common to observe a slight degree of deliberate exaggeration in many cases of a genuine work injury. And in cases of a simulated injury, the individual may only have a partial awareness that he is controlling his symptoms. The comments made about malingering in this section will refer to claims of medical conditions in which intentional motivation is the dominating element.

It is natural to keep a high index of suspicion for malingering in a compensation system. Identifying it with certainty, however, is difficult, and it is probably the most elusive condition in the system. For these reasons, it is overly suspected and underdiagnosed at the same time. While an adjuster must consider malingering when processing claims of stress injuries, it is unreasonable not to make a thorough and timely assessment when suspicions are high. When this is postponed, the case tends to become derailed in the system. Neglecting these cases prolongs their exposure to the system, and this leads invariably to delayed healing, unexpected disability and the other problems which complicate the course of industrial injuries. A major obstacle in identifying simulated conditions is the lack of a systematic method of inquiry.

Malingered disabilities cannot be detected from an absence of objective findings alone. Additionally, there must be a positive indication that an individual is deliberately producing and offering his symptoms. Unfortunately, there is no single positive indicator. Any of the findings commonly associated with malingering, such as evasiveness and dissembling, may be present in a genuine medical condition. Yet when four, five or more positive indicators are discovered, a presumptive diagnosis may be made. Drawing from clinical experience and a review of the literature, an inventory of the most reliable positive clinical indicators will be discussed.

The finding of major inconsistencies in the history and medical records is probably the most reliable sign of malingering. This is especially true when even different versions continue to proliferate long after the accident. While there are always minor discrepancies in the honest worker's description of his accident, he is still believable because the picture he paints has certain familiar qualities. The physician is impressed that the pieces of information fit well together, and there is a feeling of completeness. The course of recovery for the injury seems to be typical. This is in contrast to the history of a simulated injury which strikes the physician as being flawed by discrepancies, omissions, an atypical reaction to the accident and an unlikely clinical course.

A positive indicator reported by nonpsychiatric physicians is a distinct change in the function of the injured part during an examination. For instance, the neurologist records his impression (Tager, 1985) of marked discomfort and limited use of an extremity when it is examined, but no observed discomfort or immobility when the examination is over and the patient is getting off the table and dressing. Additionally, there is an impression the patient is deliberately altering his responses to tests of sensation, motor strength or motion. Their reports contain information that the patient jumps dramatically to simple touch and that other exaggerated responses are obvious.

In simulated psychological injuries, a positive indicator is a change in the claimant's mental status at the end of the interview. A malingering worker I once examined acted so agitated and out of touch with reality at first that I doubted we could continue. When the examination was completed, however, he was unexpectedly calm and cheerful. He chatted amicably about trivial matters and thanked me for trying to understand him. Inconsistencies in his mental status were described by other examiners. A clinical psychologist was so convinced the same worker was out of touch with reality that he cancelled the testing. Only later did the tester realize that he had been cleverly duped. Chagrin was recorded in his report as he commented that psychotic patients could be tested like anyone else and that the patient was not psychotic after the testing was cancelled. The worker had acted normal, and he talked calmly and clearly with the examiner the same way he had done at the end of my interview. Ironically, the psychologist had collected evidence of malingering without the benefit of the testing. In many cases of simulated injury, the clinician notes a dramatic normalization of behavior at the end of the examination. There is an impression that a difficult performance has been completed, and that the patient is expressing relief.

The clinical impression of dissembling is an important indicator. There is a sense that the worker is lying. His story has a contrived or rehearsed quality, or he seems to be making it up as he goes along. Instead of flowing unevenly which is the usual character of a narrative history, the dissembler's account is excessively well organized, or it contains impromptu embellishments which are introduced to impress the examiner. A valuable clue is the examiner's sense that he is being manipulated. The worker seems to be selling his story rather than offering objective information. The narrative is consistently structured to support the claimant's position that he was injured or victimized. This is in contrast to a candid narrative which is balanced and contains some information which is not in the worker's favor. Occasionally, the information offered by the worker is grossly unbelievable or there are irreconcilable elements in the history. An example is the claim of a repeated chemical exposure for which there was no treatment sought and no documentation of such an event in the medical or personnel records. Sometimes, the physician is aware that the worker's behavior in the interview is a *caricature* of a psychiatric or orthopedic condition rather than the familiar clinical picture. The features of the disorder are deliberately exaggerated according to the worker's stereotyped notions about it. Patients with genuine pain, for instance, are relatively nonvocal and withdrawn, whereas a common caricature of pain is a demonstrative claimant who yells and grimaces.

Suggestibility is another positive indicator of malingering. In this situation, the worker scrutinizes the line of questioning and behavior of the examiner for clues as to what material is making an impression. Such individuals have extraordinary skills for using the interview as a learning process for conditions about which they have no accurate foreknowledge. The examiner notices that at first, the individual is vague about his complaints but talks like an expert about his condition by the end of the interview. The degree of suggestibility can be tested by asking questions about symptoms unrelated to the injured part, or about atypical or bogus symptoms. The acknowledgement of symptoms in multiple bodily systems or migration of symptoms to adjacent areas are indicators of suggestibility and perhaps malingering. A person who answers "yes" to a question about a false symptom may have great difficulty elaborating about it if asked to do so. In contrast, a worker will offer more information about a genuine symptom without awkwardness.

Evasive behavior in the interview—an impression the worker is being uncooperative—is another positive indicator. There is a vague and infuriating quality about the way such workers describe the injury and the course of their recovery. The evasive worker ignores questions which explore the legitimacy of his claim, and he skims over his reasons for leaving past jobs. He is verbally combative when the subject of poor performance reviews is introduced, and he objects to the examiner's questions about his personal life. An uncooperative claimant may try to disarm the examiner with comments such as, "Doctor, I'll tell you anything you want to know," and then he proceeds to tell the doctor nothing. When confronted with this behavior, he apologizes profusely but his cooperation does not improve. When detailed information is requested such as employment dates, names of supervisors or time frames, the memory of the evasive worker fails. The narrative history dries up within a few moments, and the interview deteriorates into a question and answer session. Dealing with such individuals brings to mind the phrase, "like pulling teeth."

We presume that only individuals with certain enduring personality traits would deliberately contrive their disability to obtain personal benefits. Those who do usually have identifiable personality disorders, and evidence of any of these Axis II conditions should raise an adjuster's index of suspicion. The most obvious are persons who have antisocial traits. Criminal behavior, violation of the rights of others, abandonment of family, failure to pay child support, a history of fraudulent behavior, fighting, substance abuse, gambling, a nomadic life style and sexual promiscuity are the features of the antisocial personality. Often there is a family history of antisocial behavior. With this disorder, (DSM-III-R, 1987) there is always a history of occupational impairment. Such individuals are unable to sustain a good work performance, and there is a history of job changes not accounted for by type of occupation, economic cycles or seasonal fluctuations. Other signs are a violation of employer's rights, such as excessive lateness or absenteeism, lying, pilfering or embezzlement. Other work maladjustments include walking off a job without having another in sight and a similar pattern of dropping out of school or training programs without a good reason. There may be long and recurring periods of unemployment. Persons with borderline, histrionic, passive-aggressive, and paranoid traits are identified, though to a lesser extent, among those who simulate disability.

The presence of obvious incentives is a necessary indicator of a simulated disability. Common ones quickly come to mind such as money, fringe benefits, a pension, avoiding responsibility, or shifting the blame for a deficiency to someone else or to external forces. As suggested before, becoming familiar with the claimant in the totality of his life will enable a compensation professional to discover reasons why a worker might falsify an injury. Discovery of a poor work history, chronic poverty, an antisocial life style or a substance abuse problem alerts the industrial professional to the possibility of malingering.

The occurrence of a claimed injury in certain settings is yet another positive indicator of a malingered disability. Adjusters are familiar with checklists of these circumstances, and if they are kept in mind, the attempts by workers to make up an injury are often transparent. The settings involve claims made on a much-delayed basis, and when they follow a problem at work such as a poor performance review, an argument with a boss, a denial of a transfer or a failed promotion. Other suspect circumstances are the report of an injury on the first day after a weekend or scheduled vacation, or at the beginning of a shift. Positive indicators of malingering are claims of accidents which are unwitnessed by coworkers such as a fall in the restroom, in the parking lot or when the worker is off grounds on company business. The occurrence of injury claims immediately before a layoff, prior to a scheduled retirement or when seasonal work is almost done are additional indicators. Along these lines, there is an impression that the injury occurred on a "moonlighting" job or in the course of self-employment which is not covered by insurance.

The discovery of multiple positive indicators is presumptive evidence of malingering. This information can be used to weed out these claims so that the treatment of a compensable injury can be initiated without hardship to the worker.

The critical influence of false claims of injury, whether intentional or unconscious, is that delayed determination of eligibility penalizes the worker who claims a genuine injury and places him at high risk for having the complications often seen in industrial stress injuries.

Part II

Logical Management

CHAPTER NINE

Early Recognition

The most critical factor in the successful management of an industrial stress injury is early recognition. Without knowing that a worker's problems are in part or wholly psychiatric, the industrial professional will completely misunderstand the case. His decisions about the worker will be arbitrary and inappropriate, and the case will become derailed within the system. This greatly increases the risks for developing the complications seen in industrial injuries such as treatment failure, excessive disability and chronic psychological invalidism. This chapter will discuss the principles of early detection and offer clinically-oriented material about the most reliable indicators. Previous chapters have already discussed the early recognition of other clinical phenomena encountered in the industrial system such as depression (Chapter Four), secondary gain (Chapter Five), and pseudoindustrial injuries and malingering (Chapter Eight). The following material goes into detail about conversion disorder, somatoform pain disorder, post-traumatic stress disorder, adjustment disorder and organic brain syndrome.

The psychiatric literature doesn't instruct us in detail about the parameters of early recognition of industrial stress injuries. That is, how do we know when it is too late to intervene? Yet, there is a broad appreciation by compensation professionals that it is imperative to understand soon after the accident that psychological forces are playing a major role in recovery. Recognizing a psychiatric condition within weeks of the injury is usually necessary in order to have a positive impact upon its course. Because of the system's complexities, however, four to six months is a more realistic parameter. Beyond this time, the risk for complications jumps dramatically. A poor prognosis is expected for a psychiatric condition which remains undetected for more than a year.

Perhaps the psychiatric injuries overlooked the longest in a compensation system are somatoform illnesses such as a conversion disorder or a somatoform pain disorder. The principles of early recognition can well be illustrated by retrospective study of cases in which a diagnosis of one of these disorders was eventually established.

Delayed healing and prolonged recovery of an apparent physical injury are probably the most reliable early signs that psychological factors are influencing the course of the case. Physicians recognize that the body heals in a generally predictable period of time. A worker who is still totally disabled four to five months after suffering a mild back sprain probably has an emotional component to his pain and stiffness if not a full-blown somatoform disorder. Experience suggests that marked dysfunction in the worker's domestic life is the next most useful clue. Its significance may not be readily apparent. Ordinarily, an active person who is disabled by a back strain wants to return to normal function as quickly as possible. He pushes the limits set by his doctor. He ignores the recommendation for bedrest, lifts too much and breaks the rules altogether by mowing his lawn or playing a round of golf. To the dismay of his spouse, he limps to his car one morning with a full toolbox and goes to work two weeks early. His eagerness to resume normal activities may lead to a setback and a prolonged recovery, but there can be no doubt about his motivation to work.

On the other hand, a similarly injured worker who cannot get out of bed by himself, prepare a snack, perform the most menial of household chores, answer the telephone, drive a car, or otherwise lift a finger on his own behalf probably has a somatoform disorder. An inventory of a worker's domestic and personal functioning after an injury may reveal some of these unexpected impairments. The worker's helpless behavior is an attempt to manipulate his wife, children, friends and employer to lower their expectations for him to be self-sufficient and productive. Near-invalidism at home may be the earliest indication that the worker's symptoms are determined by psychological factors rather than a bodily injury.

Industrial professionals must discern early in recovery that a worker is responding poorly or not at all to treatment, and that even time has no apparent healing effect. A paradoxical response to treatment is a valuable early clue. Treatment ordinarily expected to reduce a patient's pain, instead, makes him feel more uncomfortable. This response suggests the worker is not eager to give up his symptoms and that psychogenic factors are at work. During this period there are characteristic remarks from the worker such as, "None of the doctors have ever helped me," or "It just gets worse and worse everyday."

That an alleged physical injury is really a psychiatric problem can be determined early-on by a characteristic pattern of reporting in the medical records. In the case of a conversion disorder, for instance, the notes of the very first doctors who attended the injured worker may reflect puzzlement about the genuineness of the problem. Subjective findings far exceed objective ones. In many such cases the observation of "no findings" is clearly documented, or the doctor may choose his words carefully to merely imply his doubt concerning his patient's complaints. The doctor may record his impression of inconsistencies in the history or the findings. Bewilderment or disbelief that a fairly mundane accident could have a catastrophic result may be expressed in these early files.

The injurious events held responsible for these conditions are typically minor ones. They are the accidents which would be expected to disable most workers for a day or two and several weeks at the most. Commonly they include a slip-and-fall accident, being struck by a small falling object or a lifting incident. The setting of the accident may provide the critical clue that psychogenic factors underlie a worker's disability. Early recognition is facilitated if it is noted that the injury occurred in close association with an argument with a coworker, a poor performance review, counselling by a manager or denial of a transfer. Major threats to a worker's career or pension also trigger these conditions. A failed promotion, forced early retirement, geographical move or receiving notice the company is a target of a corporate "take-over" are sometimes the only explanation for a failed treatment. Knowledge of a concurrent trauma in the worker's personal life, such as a lost relationship, is often the earliest indicator that the patient has a conversion disorder instead of a physically deranged hand. Strong evidence of a potential or existing secondary gain issue should suggest a somatoform disorder.

Within a few weeks or months of the injury, the medical records of these workers contain a growing collection of information to strengthen the diagnosis of a psychiatric disorder rather than an orthopedic or neurologic injury. There are numerous consultations and diagnostic tests, multiple forms of treatment hospitalization or referral to distant clinics. Subjective symptoms dominate the clinical picture, and there is a growing awareness that objective findings cannot be reproduced and are absent. The records make no mention of a definite diagnosis, and often there is a long list of diagnoses. Commonly, these patients are given a false diagnosis such as "functional overlay," "fasciitis" or "post-traumatic syndrome." Various kinds of physical therapy or self-administrated exercise regimes are useless, or they aggravate the condition. The patient isn't getting any better, and the doctors are confused.

With no other way to feel useful to their patient, they prescribe a large variety of pain-killers, antispasmodics and anti-inflammatory agents, none of which has any lasting benefit. Eventually the treating doctor cannot help noticing that the patient is emotionally upset because of his physical problems, and he prescribes additional medications such as hypnotics, tranquilizers and antidepressants. These drugs have many side effects, and the clinical picture is further clouded. Some patients become addicted to them. With confusion growing, the rationale for continuing these drugs is lost. The course of these disorders is now characterized by a chronic state of impasse in which the patient continues to come in monthly for meaningless office visits and receive useless prescriptions for treatment. There is a growing awareness by compensation professionals that nothing is happening in the case, each progress note reads like the last, and recovery has come to a halt. This kind of stagnation in a patient's recovery is highly suggestive of a somatoform disorder.

The pattern and nature of the physical complaints suggest the real nature of the condition. Obvious are symptoms which violate anatomical reality, or which cannot be explained by physiological principles. There are more subtle patterns, such as symptoms which migrate to nearby areas or shift back and forth from one extremity to the other. Extension of complaints to other bodily systems is also a good early indicator of a psychogenic problem. For example, a worker with unexplained shoulder pain begins to complain about dizziness, shortness of breath, a poor memory and soreness of his hips. The appearance of entirely new problems several weeks or months after the injury is an early clue. A sudden worsening of the original complaint is a common event, especially when the doctor is about to return his patient to work.

An additional area to explore is the worker's personality characteristics. Only certain individuals develop these disorders. Traits of dependency, psychological immaturity and hysteria predispose a worker to a psychogenic pain disorder. Many lack the control mechanisms for coping with intense emotion, and they are prone to feeling bodily aches when under stress. Many people evidently lack a capacity to perceive their feelings. Disturbing emotion is always experienced in the form of physical pain. This tendency is additionally found among individuals who have a lack of education, a poor work record, a disorganized life style or a background in which somatization of emotional problems is a strong cultural trait.

Evidence of suggestibility is sometimes the earliest indicator of a conversion disorder. If asked if they have certain symptoms, such claimants say "yes" to all questions, or they will circle all the items on written tests which suggest pathology to them, even though they failed to mention having these problems initially. If an inventory of symptoms is offered to suggestible persons, it is common for them to simply reply, "I have all of that." On one occasion I asked a worker if he had certain aches and pains only to hear, "Now that you bring it up, my whole life hurts." Offering a survey of human pathology to a suggestible worker opens up opportunities for using illness to manipulate the system and cannot be done without the risk of generating additional claims of injury.

The first principle of early recognition then, is careful monitoring of the case from the first days, weeks and months of the accident with an eye for certain tell-tale signs, some obvious and some subtle. Other clues are specific, and still others exist only as patterns or trends in the case, or as small bits of information, each having little significance by itself. Any suggestive information should lead to a careful perusal of the evidence for additional clues. The time for psychiatric assessment or testing is early during recovery when these clues begin to crop up.

The second principle is suggested by the slowness with which information is disseminated in a multi-party health care system. Being the first to learn about a problem is a position which allows options. Depending on the interests of the discovering party, information can be shared at once, or it can be ignored, giving it an uncertain fate in the channels of communication. If the interest is quickly returning the worker to his job, sharing is the option of choice. The tendency for stress injuries to have a downhill course is assured by a failure to disclose psychiatric issues. For the reasons elaborated upon in this book, lengthy involvement in a compensation system increases the worker's risk for complications, and limiting this exposure is in his best interest.

The option to withhold knowledge of a stress injury may be exercised by some as loss-reducing measure, hoping that the injury will remain undetected by others. This action is based on an assumption that the problem will disappear spontaneously. Experience suggests otherwise, and ignoring it to save money is an example of false economy. Side-stepping the stress components of an injury merely increases the extent of the worker's involvement in the system. As medical complications delay recovery, costs are expected to spiral. The second principal of early recognition is sharing the discovery of a stress injury with the other players in the system at once. Applying one without the other will not benefit anyone.

Timely recognition of other common stress-related disorders can be facilitated by knowing the natural history of these conditions and their early manifestations. The diagnostic criteria for these psychiatric conditions are set forth clearly in DSM-III-R and will not be repeated here. Anticipating their *associated* features is also helpful. A certain percentage of persons who have been exposed to extreme psychological stress develop the familiar signs and symptoms of a post-traumatic stress disorder. While the onset is often delayed for months, there are some very early indicators, the most notable of which is an aversion response.

This is essentially an avoidance of dangers which have been unrealistically magnified following a physical injury or psychologically traumatic event. In the thinking of the victim, reinjury is inevitable upon reexposure to the same danger or a similar one. In most accidents or close-calls, temporary avoidance of the hazard is a normal and expected reaction, but sometimes the aversion becomes a permanent feature of a person's life. An explosion victim, for example, makes no attempt to reenter the plant, and a toolmaker who sustains a hand injury is too frightened to operate machinery again. A phobic aversion which is still present six months after an accident will probably persist.

Other indicators of a stress disorder are frequent recollections of the accident. They take the form of recurring nightmares and images of the injury scene which intrude upon the worker during waking hours. In this situation, the emotional shock triggered by the accident fails to subside, and long afterward the worker experiences the accident as if it had occurred only hours or days before. As in the case of somatoform disorders, it is important to inquire about the worker's personal life. The emotional numbing and reduced involvement so characteristic of a stress disorder can be detected early by asking questions about his relationships with family members, friends and coworkers.

Victims of harassment seldom develop the full-blown picture of a post-traumatic stress disorder. However, they often complain of a phobic aversion for returning to a job setting where they will have contact with the perpetrator. Even the prospect for having a chance encounter is so terrifying that many harassment victims will remain disabled until this risk is eliminated. As noted in Chapter

Two, individuals who become victims of this kind of abuse have a special vulnerability related to an inhibition for expressing negative emotion. Their dread for reencountering the person who harassed them is actually a fear of having their own reactive anger come to the surface. In large part, this is the same dread for showing anger which had upset their psychological equilibrium to begin with. Early recognition of this aversion is critical to successful management of harassment injuries.

When work disrupts an individual's psychological equilibrium, there is apparently no limit to the variety and number of emotional or physical symptoms this can produce. The most common diagnosis associated with occupational stress is an *adjustment disorder.* DSM-III-R defines an adjustment disorder as "a maladaptive reaction to an identifiable psychosocial stressor, or stressors, that occurs, within three months after onset of the stressor, and has persisted for no longer than six months. The maladaptive nature of the reaction is indicated either by impairment in occupational (including school) functioning or in usual social activities or relationships with others or by symptoms that are in excess of a normal and expectable reaction to the stressor. The disturbance is not merely one instance of a pattern of overreaction to stress or an exacerbation of one of the mental disorders previous described in the manual."

In industry, the stressor may be a specific problem such as a demotion or an ongoing one such as a low back syndrome. Following an injury, for example, a person normally experiences some degree of emotional instability. Predictably, there are anxious and depressive symptoms, and he will use more immature ways of coping with the external world. The diagnosis of adjustment disorder should be made only when there is clear-cut evidence that a worker's responses to his injury are maladaptive or unexpected. Adjustment disorder should not be confused with normal grieving which accompanies a major loss of health. In this process, the worker experiences temporary periods of anger, frustration and depression which are necessary ingredients in his recovery.

While assessing a worker's psychological responses to his injuries, it is difficult to draw a line between normal and abnormal. However, a worker's behavior can be viewed as unequivocally maladaptive if he fails to make an adequate effort to rehabilitate himself or acts self-destructively. This diagnosis would apply if he causes himself to be additionally injured, fails to keep appointments or sabotages his treatment regime. The same is true if he develops a substance abuse problem, becomes a near-invalid at home, alienates his family or becomes suicidal. This diagnosis can be used if the worker has certain symptoms which clearly impair his functioning or threaten his well being. A marked sleep impairment prevents someone from getting adequate rest, and a large weight gain threatens a person's physical health. An inability to focus thoughts for more than a few minutes prevents an injured worker from participating in a retraining program. Anxiety attacks have a disruptive effect on day-to-day activities, and a severely depressed mood may destroy a worker's capacity to envisage a future for himself.

With these guidelines in mind, a compensation professional can make a timely differentiation between an adjustment disorder and normal reactions to an injury. Monitoring the injured worker's progress in this way will commonly be rewarded by the early detection of this condition which, in turn, may require psychiatric treatment or a change in management tactics.

If severe anxiety attacks reduce a back-injured worker's ability to cope with pain, he may need psychiatric treatment before his condition can be accurately assessed and treated. Or a structured retraining program will have to be postponed until a worker with severe depression and an inability to concentrate receives antidepressant medication. A worker with an iatrogenic substance abuse problem will have to undergo detoxification and drug rehabilitation before treatment of the original industrial injury can resume. And a worker who is undermining his treatment and recovery may require the joint efforts of his family, doctor, attorney, adjustor and rehabilitation counselor. A worker who is psychologically inhibited from working may require psychotherapy before he can return to his job. With a way to detect adjustment disorders early, the industrial professional has a tool with which he can make intelligent alterations of his management strategy.

Too often, organic brain syndromes remain undetected in the case loads of the industrial professional. After a major accident such as a fall or a vehicular collision, mild brain damage is overlooked when there are more compelling injuries such as a major fracture or life-threatening blood loss. Subtle intellectual impairments may not be detected until much later. Clinically, mild dementia cannot be easily differentiated from common psychiatric disorders. The diagnosis is further obscured by the ability of brain-injured persons to compensate for their limitations or partially disguise them. The most reliable early sign is a memory deficit for recent events. Recalling the distant past is remarkably intact. Forgetfulness in daily functioning is common. Such persons are forever losing track of where they placed their car keys, wallet, tools, notes or other personal items. They create hazards by leaving burning cigarettes around the house or pots on the stove. They cannot remember appointments or other commitments unless they are entered in a calendar. Without written lists or the assistance of family members, they are unable to function.

The failure of recent memory function is usually intermittent and unpredictable, and this has a highly disruptive effect upon everyday activities. Frequently such persons forget what they are talking about in conversations and fill in the gaps with extraneous material. Retention of new material is nearly impossible. Becoming disoriented while driving, even in their own community, is common, and such workers cannot transport themselves to unfamiliar medical centers without making a trial run ahead of time. In most cases of brain dysfunction, there is obvious occupational dysfunction. A carpenter may forget how to perform routine tasks, and a person in a position of management may appear to colleagues as grossly disorganized and inappropriate.

In addition to intellectual impairments, personality changes can frequently be detected soon after the injury. Poor impulse control, temper tantrums and a tendency to cry for no reason are common manifestations of mild dementia. There is a loss of tolerance for the ordinary irritations which were handled before with ease. For example, a person who loved dogs may yell and throw objects at them whenever they bark. The range of interpersonal involvement is narrowed, and there may be permanent reduction in their sexual functioning. A deterioration of dress and grooming may be noticeable to family members, and there is a repetitive, stereotyped manner of behaving and speaking. Enduring personality traits are seen in greater relief, and characteristic disturbances in interpersonal relationships may occur. They may completely ignore previously enjoyed activities, and those around notice a pervasive constriction of functioning and movements.

Early recognition of dementia may be accomplished by having a knowledge of the pattern of clinical findings outlined above and a high level of suspicion in certain cases. Obviously, these include all major injuries, head injuries, falls, automobile collisions, and accidents in which there is a history of unconsciousness. Detecting organic brain syndromes early will greatly facilitate their management. Since recovery is virtually complete two years after the injury, there is an aspect of predictability about the course of these conditions. Residual intellectual impairments, especially a memory deficit and poor retention, limit the usefulness of vocational rehabilitation.

Logical management of industrial stress injuries depends first upon detecting them within weeks of the injury. This enables an industrial professional to exert early control over a case in order to prevent the numerous problems which commonly interrupt the worker's recovery. The following chapters will discuss other important ingredients of a logical management. These include a time-tested treatment strategy, a systematic way of analyzing a case load, and ways to prevent complications.

CHAPTER TEN

The Facilitative Process

To make effective decisions about an industrial stress injury, the therapist, case manager or other professional must recognize the particular areas of a worker's functioning which are impaired, and then decide what specific assistance is needed. In the simplest instance, a depressed worker may be too fatigued from lack of sleep or distracted by emotional pain to perform his job. Or a labile person may be too irritable to relate normally to co-workers. Remedies to overcome these common symptoms come to mind, such as prescribing a leave of absence or medication. However, applying them in the industrial system may be useless and even harmful. One of the peculiar features of compensation injuries is an overrepresentation of individuals within the system with impaired problem-solving ability. Whether by default—people habitually lacking in resources to fall back upon—or because of maladaptive character traits, the deck is stacked against the industrial professional.

It can be seen that the vulnerabilities which caused a worker to suffer a stress-related injury in the first place are carried over into the benefit delivery system. These are the same traits which are expected to interact maladaptively with the forces encountered there. Any action taken by a professional to treat or rehabilitate an injured worker must take such susceptibilities into account. Perhaps the most common forms of behavior encountered in this system are helplessness and excessive dependency upon others. There are several reasons for this. Persons with these traits naturally gravitate to a compensation system. Illness or injury normally has a psychologically regressive effect, and the system tends to place people in a dependent position. Because helpless patterns of behaving are so pervasive in the system and the risks for reinforcing them so high, the overriding principle of managing stress disorders is the use of a facilitative approach.

To facilitate means to ease or make less difficult. For the professional helper it defines a certain stance taken with a person who is struggling with a psychological illness or other personal dilemma. A facilitative approach involves more in the way of clearing obstacles, enabling, empowering, clarifying and confronting than serving, nurturing, taking over, giving medication or providing solutions. It requires an attitude of expectancy on the part of the professional helper who consistently gives messages to his patient that he is capable of finding ways to solve his own problems. This is opposed to taking action on the patient's behalf and providing services such as advice or recommendations. The essential feature of the facilitative approach is that of placing the responsibility for an individual's problems squarely on his shoulders.

Pressures to shift this burden to the therapist or other professional are always resisted. The facilitative process is analogous to a tennis game in which a winning strategy is to try to keep the ball in the other person's court. This "game plan" has advantages in helping anyone who has problems, and it is practically mandatory for dealing with individuals whose coping style involves excess use of passive behavior. The facilitative process forces a person to discover and make use of unused resources. Whatever solution he finds will be of his own design, suited to meet his unique needs and one which affords control over his destiny. Few people would seriously try to solve someone else's problems or conduct another's life. No mature parent believes he can be responsible for his child's homework or choose his friends. Most of us have no difficulty with the concept that we must be responsible for our own welfare and that entrusting it to someone else is a folly.

This principle must be applied when trying to help a disabled person get back on his feet. There is a misconception that physicians have powers to heal their patients. Only the body can heal itself, and the orthopedic surgeon who places a pin in the fractured leg of his patient is providing a facilitative service. While it is true that his patient plays a passive role when he receives anesthesia and submits to surgery, his role thereafter is an active and responsible one. The patient facilitates healing by protecting his cast and postponing a return to normal activity until his doctor says he is ready. In the treatment of psychiatric conditions, the responsibility for making changes or resolving conflicts is left to the patient. Nothing is done to place the patient in a passive position such as offering advice, making recommendations or providing remedies. Assisting the patient directly may be a temptation for the industrial professional, but advice and solutions are not facilitative.

Rather than address the worker's specific deficiencies, such "help" backfires by reinforcing the same ineffective coping behavior which contributed to his difficulties to begin with. The message received by the worker is that he is incapable of solving his own problems, let alone understand them, and that others know what is best. The way out of his dilemma is to place himself in the industrial professional's hands. In the thinking of the dependent personality, such counseling means his problems are essentially solved. So often, it reinforces a literal interpretation of the employer's responsibility, which is to "cure" him of the effects of the injury. Unfortunately, such persons lose sight of the actuality that this is a legal concept and has no counterpart in real life (or in an effective psychotherapy.)

It is easy to forget that dependent persons have always permitted others to direct their lives. Seldom is it appreciated that this is not left to chance but is manipulated. This is accomplished by defaulting on their responsibilities at every opportunity. Helpless behavior compels concerned people to take over and make decisions for them. There is a paradox in helplessness, and that is its power. Individuals with these traits are skilled at coercing others to do precisely what they want, and they can be regarded as having a special faculty. Experience teaches us that their strengths go well beyond this, and that even the most pitiful-appearing person who begs for relief has far greater resources than he shows. Only a facilitative approach will defeat this manipulation and enable the individual to extricate himself from his plight.

The facilitative process is applied by a psychotherapist who focuses on the patient's *responses* to events around him rather than the *events* themselves. When the worker complains about the frustrations of being in a compensation system, the therapist shows his patient how he expects too much from the system and uses inaction in an attempt to meet his needs. How effective the patient is in managing his situation is kept to the forefront. The therapist is nonfacilitative if he is overly sympathetic and allies himself with the patient's dilemma. Each time the patient tries to shift his responsibilities to the therapist, this maneuver is pointed out. There are demands for action or answers. The therapist is facilitative if he points out realistically that providing direct services would be counterproductive. Doing so would merely make him dependent upon the therapist for solutions, and the hole he finds himself in would be dug even deeper.

The facilitative process begins during the first sessions. Commonly, the stress-injured worker wants resolution of his dilemma *before* returning to his job. Instead of agreeing to this arrangement, a facilitative therapist expects his patient to involve himself in the external world as a condition of treatment. The sessions can then be used to clarify problems which occur in here-and-now situations. The nonfacilitative therapist agrees to a get-well-first treatment and finds himself in the absurd situation of dealing with distant conflicts which seem more abstract than real. Even if the patient is too dysfunctional to meet this condition at once, the issue is kept to the forefront of therapy. When the patient has unrealistic attitudes such as viewing treatment as a "lifeline," the facilitative therapist challenges this viewpoint and introduces the notion that only the patient can lift himself from his dilemma. It is common for workers to feel greatly victimized. The facilitative therapist communicates an appreciation of his patient's anguish but points out at every opportunity that he is doing nothing constructive to disentangle himself from his problems. A nonfacilitative therapist listens excessively to these complaints and fails to show his patient that more constructive actions are being overlooked. The issues brought to the therapy sessions, even compelling ones, are not allowed to take priority over the establishment of a facilitative treatment. In this process, what is happening in the therapy is constantly monitored.

The questions the therapist must ask himself are: Am I promoting self-sufficiency or reinforcing dependency? Or in the tennis game analogy: Am I trying to place the ball in the other person's court?

For reasons already set forth, an industrial injury may be the greatest crisis faced by a person in his lifetime. The longer he remains in the system, the greater is the risk of suffering a crippling complication. An industrial helper facilitates recovery if he enables his patient or client to see that he is up against some discouraging realities. There is an obligation, for instance, to point out that considering the self-serving forces at work within the system that he, the injured worker, is in the best position to determine what is best for his own welfare. To facilitate recovery, he convinces the worker that taking charge of his destiny and limiting his dependence upon the system are in his best interests. At the very beginning, the industrial practitioner sets the stage for surviving in the compensation system. To recover, the worker will have to reach back and discover unused resources. Secondary gain behavior must be confronted and clarified. Adversive treatment conditions and bias about psychiatric conditions are pointed out as pitfalls which may slow his recovery. The worker must be shown that he places himself in jeopardy by sitting back and waiting for someone else to act, or for his luck to change. He may have to work it all out for himself.

Illustrating this process, a general practitioner who was skilled at managing industrial injuries informed his patients that they alone were in a position to bring about recovery and a return to productive life. On hearing this, most felt some empowerment and became more aggressive in their treatment and rehabilitation programs. Others reacted with disappointment or anger. The doctor properly understood these responses as a positive sign, an indication his patients were mourning the loss of the "powerful other person" whom they had imagined would bring their suffering to an end. Still others reacted with denial and disbelief. The doctor gently but firmly put off other treatment concerns until his patient better understood the reality of his circumstances. Those strongly resistant to the notion of helping themselves were asked: "You mean, if there were no system, you would do nothing?" This addressed the main deficiency in the thinking of passive individuals that they couldn't survive without the intervention of a more powerful force. The doctor facilitated the recovery of his patients by scrapping this idea and encouraging them to assume the responsibility for their lives.

Examples of a nonfacilitative approach are treatments which promise to do certain things for the patient, such as a hands-on remedy, a "proven method," medication, or other approaches which place the patient in a passive or receptive position. Like all nonfacilitative interventions, the relief afforded is temporary; when treatment stops, symptoms reappear. In the industrial system, promises are offered when there are pressures to take action and an enabling strategy is overlooked. The rationale is that doing something is better than doing nothing. Unfortunately, such action is not merely perfunctory. It may have real traumatizing effects. In the process, the patient is systematically trained to act even more helpless and dependent. With his resources frozen, the worker no longer struggles against his disease, which is allowed to progress and become entrenched. Chronic psychological invalidism is a common result.

By way of illustration, I was asked to evaluate Curtis, a single bus driver in his late twenties who had been absent from his job for more than a year because of typical stress symptoms. Curtis suffered a dislocated shoulder and rib fractures when his bus struck a large truck in a chain-reaction accident during a rainstorm. Referral for psychiatric treatment was made by his orthopedic surgeon when Curtis began to hyperventilate during an office visit. The therapist learned of other symptoms such as stomach distress, vomiting, headaches, shaky feelings and fears about returning to his route. His anxious symptoms were triggered by the doctor's comment that Curtis would soon be released for work. Psychiatric treatment was recommended and accepted by Curtis, who was baffled by his reactions and had bills piling up. After a year of psychotherapy, however, he did not feel ready to resume working.

Evaluation revealed that Curtis had grown up in a disrupted family and that he always felt anxious and unsure of himself. He denied having major problems in school or in his social life. Until the doctor talked about releasing him to work, Curtis was prepared to return to his bus-driving job despite the usual stressors such as rowdy teenagers, drunk passengers, heavy traffic and hassles with supervisors. Background revealed that in his early teen years Curtis accidently scratched the eye of a playmate in a swimming pool. This resulted in a hemorrhage which partially blinded his friend. Years after the accident Curtis struggled with guilty feelings and concerns about injuring someone. He avoided trying out for high school sports because of these fears. It was evident that Curtis was struggling with a complex intertwining of past and current psychological conflicts which had immobilized him since the accident. He dreaded facing his supervisor and the day when he would have to account for his role in the accident. Ordinary job pressures Curtis had handled in the past were now expected to be overwhelming. His problem wasn't an uncommon one and should not have posed any treatment difficulties for an experienced therapist. Resolution was expected within a relatively short time, but somehow psychotherapy had gotten onto the wrong track.

The reason was easy to find. His treatment was non-facilitative. The therapist believed his job was to comfort and protect his fearful patient. He was overly sympathetic when Curtis talked about the frustrations of his job and supported his position that driving a bus was a hazardous occupation. Curtis learned he would not be released until all his fears were allayed. He savored the treatment sessions and made repeated references to his therapist as his "mentor." Instead of encouraging action and self-sufficiency, the therapist had relieved Curtis of the responsibility for his problems and placed him in a passive position. The specific psychological conflicts disabling Curtis were not being addressed. In this process, Curtis was losing rather than gaining self-confidence, and any mention of returning to work caused his anxiety to resurface.

It is not difficult to envision a facilitative therapy for

Curtis in which self-confidence is promoted by placing the burden for resolution on his shoulders. Rather than treat him as if he were a child, the therapist would facilitate adult problem-solving behavior. Early in the treatment, Curtis would be expected to find a way to return to work and to account for his role in the accident. Some hard realities would be faced in therapy. Curtis would be encouraged to talk about the increase in anxiety he expects to feel while driving again, and when he encounters road conditions which remind him of the accident. It may be necessary for Curtis to learn that his reactions to the collision were influenced by the accident in his teenage years. Unless Curtis could make some steps in this direction soon after his dilemma surfaced, he was at risk for developing a chronic illness. Regardless of the type of psychotherapy preferred by the mental health professional, a facilitative style is especially useful in countering the passivity, inaction and avoidance of responsibility which is seen commonly in industrial injuries.

Sometimes, this idea can be taken a step further. In cases where the worker's recovery is mired in impasse, the failure of the industrial system suggests a solution. Stepping outside of the system may be the only way for a worker to regain control of his life, and the industrial practitioner who facilitates this move has performed a valuable service. In psychiatry, "no treatment" is always a viable alternative to treatment, and the facilitative therapist makes this clear during the first visits. With a little ingenuity, a different viewpoint or mobilizing unused resources, many seemingly impossible problems can be resolved. This approach was used in the case of a machinist I once saw who had been disabled for several years with a low back syndrome. Several surgeries had failed to relieve his pain, and he faced an uncertain future. Over the years, he had been offered a considerable amount of rehabilitation and treatment services. The referral was made for treatment of depression and mental clouding. When I suggested that perhaps the compensation system had nothing left to offer and that he had overlooked the strategy of working out his own solution, my patient was startled at first but felt empowered to come up with an idea. Determined not to live out his life as an invalid, and convinced he could be at work with pain as well as stay at home, he contacted virtually every potential employer within commute distance and laid out his predicament. His efforts were rewarded by a position as a shop supervisor with a flexible work format.

The case manager can monitor the facilitative process by asking if the professional interventions in the case will reinforce passive behavior or promote self-sufficiency. Keeping the tennis analogy in mind, he must ask whether or not the therapist or rehabilitation counselor is trying to keep the ball in the worker's court.

CHAPTER ELEVEN

Management by Asking the Right Questions

Intelligent management of an industrial stress injury depends upon understanding the case as a whole before the first decision is made about it. Developing a meaningful overview requires more than administrative problem-solving and shuffling of paper. In the everyday process of managing a case load, it is easy to forget that the injured worker remains an individual, someone whose life has been disrupted and who usually has few resources to fall back upon. Months and years after an accident, it can be overlooked that a person's life will be dominated by the influences of the industrial system, a myriad of forces seldom seen in non-work cases. The worker has little knowledge of this system or power to control it. For the industrial practitioner, it is not enough to realize that his actions will have an important impact on the worker's welfare. The factors which determine the recovery of an injured worker are specific, and they are always multiple and interactive. A management decision will make sense only in the context of all these determining factors and when there is an appreciation of how they operate together. Identifying them quickly and knowing how they interact to affect the worker is the fundamental task in managing industrial stress injuries. Otherwise, there is no rational guideline for making decisions about the case each step along the way as it moves through the benefit delivery system.

Unfortunately, there is little time for doing this. The

natural history of stress injuries is for something to go wrong during recovery. Soon after the injury, the case is all too often nudged onto a destructive course. The first decisions are the most important ones. The administrator must remind himself that he is operating in a dynamic, interactive system, one in which a vulnerable person will react to his decision and the turn of events influenced by it, in a highly individualistic way. If the adjuster, doctor or lawyer has taken the time to familiarize himself with this interplay, his management efforts will be rewarded by a remarkable degree of predictability. Without this foreknowledge, his decisions will be arbitrary. He will flail about and increase the worker's risks for developing some of the dreaded complications seen so frequently in these cases. Because there are many influences such as the worker's personality, the hazards of the system, and secondary gain issues, a systematic approach is necessary.

One way is to make an inventory of the factors which critically influence the case by asking the right questions. The product of this inquiry is a *formulation* or *psychological explanation* of the case. This is a written capsule or brief, recorded in a few sentences, which describes the central conflicts which upset the worker's psychological equilibrium and caused him to express the disturbance outwardly as symptoms such as panic or depression. It summarizes the interplay of environmental stressors and the person's susceptibilities to them. A formulation is an expression of the repetitive ways an individual reacts to events taking place about him (Perry, 1987), and it is not expected to change greatly. Because of its stable nature, the formulation can serve as a road map for treatment and other actions taken by compensation professionals. As a reliable reminder of how an injured worker is expected to respond to decisions made about him, it can be placed in a conspicuous place in his medical or rehabilitation file. When changes occur in the environment or the way the worker copes with them, the formulation can be updated and modified.

Similar to a psychiatric diagnosis, a formulation is short, specific and oversimplified. It goes beyond a diagnosis by providing detailed information about the patient's expected way of operating in his environment. It contains practical knowledge of how the individual will cope with the rigors of the industrial system as he recuperates. A brief conceptualization is a useful management tool in industrial cases where the factors determining the course of the illnesses are numerous to begin with and tend to proliferate with time.

Amidst these disruptive forces, the formulation is a buffer or a stabilizing force. Manipulations by the worker or the other parties can be resisted, and abrupt changes in management tactics can be warded off. The mental health worker can use the formulation to direct his efforts logically and consistently. From the beginning, the mental health professional is advantaged by having a guide for his patient's problems. Too often psychotherapists are excessively passive and offer narrowly-focused, stereotyped responses to material initiated by the patient. The scope of therapy is limited to what the patient brings to each session or what he can understand about his illness on his own. This verbal hand holding accomplishes nothing, and eventually, the psychologically-injured worker senses the therapist doesn't understand his deficiencies or decides that psychiatric treatment doesn't work in the first place. On the other hand, by conceptualizing his patient's problems using a formulation, the therapist has a systematic method to be helpful rather than having to rely on intuition or his patient for conducting the treatment.

Psychotherapists are not the only ones who can use a dynamic explanation of the case. Attorneys, adjusters, rehabilitation counselors and surgical specialists can better understand their client by writing a synopsis. They can view the individual's hostility, helplessness or failure to comply with recommendations as reactive behavior which is understandable and predictable in the light of the forces within the system and his enduring behavioral traits. This appreciation can help them accept the worker's symptoms without being judgmental. It can inspire new strategies for assisting him.

Writing down a dynamic formulation has many advantages. It encourages serious thought about clinical material. More than simply expanding on an impression, the writing process forces a detailed, piece by piece study of a psychological dilemma. While forming the puzzle, the nature of missing pieces or omissions will be apparent. Some bits of information will never fit, and presumptions about the case may have to be changed. The written formulation humanizes the case, especially if the worker's name is used. It reminds a busy compensation professional that the chart on his desk represents a unique human dilemma, not merely a claimant, for instance, with a low back syndrome. Making a written capsule of the case is a valuable trouble-shooting tool in a case which is not making any progress. The reasons for the impasse can be spotted. The presence of this document in a conspicuous place on the chart is a recurring reminder of the strategy to follow when making decisions about that individual. It serves as a guide for judging the actions taken by other players in the system. Having it readily available can alert someone to a destructive element in the case. Monitoring the worker's recovery is eased, as certain patterns, crises or turning points can be foreseen and promptly diagnosed. In this application, the dynamic formulation can suggest the most useful time for reexamination. New information can be tested for its validity and the formulation modified if there are recent developments.

In the field of psychiatry, the term "dynamics" is

often used interchangeably with "psychodynamics," which is more traditional. Psychodynamics refers to the mental determinants of behavior or illness which therapists rely heavily upon to understand and treat their patients. Other influences such as age, education, life circumstances or a concurrent physical illness are "nondynamic" determinants. For practical purposes in this book, the use of the term "dynamics" refers to all the determinants of a worker's behavior, whether psychological, situational or one of the critically influencing factors outlined in earlier chapters. Understanding the dynamics of an industrial case simply means that the major forces which shape the course of his recovery are identified, and there is an appreciation of how these forces operate together to influence the worker's reactions.

As suggested, the dynamic formulation can be a few sentences, enough to identify the main issues. It can be something simple like advising that, "Ms. Allen is off work with a severe depression because of harassment and will not return to her job unless she is protected from further contact with her coworker. Depression is less an issue than the presence of the perpetrator in the office. Ms. Allen learned that she will not be transferred." This capsule clearly maps out the correct management strategy, which is to alert interested parties, mainly her company, that job modification is necessary. Instead, if the focus is on treatment and the parties are waiting for the psychiatrist to sign Ms. Allen's release, the problem at work would be ignored, and the wait would be a long one.

Or it can be more elaborate, as in the case of a manager who was able to function adequately for many years in the same job but developed disabling anxiety when promoted and given heavier responsibilities: "After Mr. Brown was placed on leave, he became very depressed and withdrawn. He is too depressed to go back right away. He recently sought psychiatric treatment. Mr. Brown grew up in a disrupted family and as a teenager probably struggled with untreated depression. In college, he was a good student but received counseling for anxiety attacks which occurred when he took examinations. Treatment apparently helped. In his department, Mr. Brown was considered a good worker but was always quiet and lacked ambition. He held the same job for 15 years. The promotion was offered passively. His family life is stable, and he has no other problems. Mr. Brown needs time and treatment."

The formulation advises that Mr. Brown has a good work record and a history of having used psychotherapy as a young man to overcome a difficult problem. It should suggest to an experienced professional that with time, adequate treatment and rebuilding of his confidence, Mr. Brown's prognosis is good. While the capsule doesn't state this in so many words, it paints a useful picture of a basically stable person who was psychologically vulnerable to the greater pressures of his new job. In the meantime, Mr. Brown is grieving his losses—his mental health and his failed assignment. The formulation advises that he would react tentatively at first to the assistance offered in the industrial system, but he would ultimately make good use of its services and return to a productive life.

This capsule deliberately has an optimistic tone and suggests that, unlike Ms. Allen's case, secondary gain issues are absent. It encourages an attitude of patience with a need to respond generously when Mr. Brown is feeling better and ready to put more effort into his recovery. This dynamic formulation is simplistic, considering that a complete explanation of Mr. Brown's dilemma would be rich and detailed. But in the industrial system, such a document would not serve any practical purpose. The capsule as suggested above is quite useful. It reminds his employer and the adjuster not to infuriate Mr. Brown by calling to ask when he is coming back to work. Such impatient inquiries would reinforce his sense of failure and prolong recovery. The formulation guides them toward a waiting and supportive strategy. This worker has suffered a severe psychological injury which is much like a major bone fracture and requires time to heal. The capsule reminds the occupational nurse, for instance, that the employee with depression is no different, and telephone calls placed to Mr. Brown should be nondemanding and show genuine concern.

Creating a formulation requires discovery of the determinants of an injured worker's recovery and an understanding of how they operate together to facilitate or impede his progress. The systematic way to accomplish this is twofold. The first step is to ask the right questions. The second is to use the answers to create a mental impression of how the worker is interacting with the system to recuperate from his injuries. This process is analogous to discovering the pieces of a complicated puzzle and fitting them together until an image forms. The emerging picture should make sense to the industrial professional in the light of his knowledge and experience. If the pieces fail to fit together and the picture is unfamiliar, then more questions will have to be asked.

The first two questions concern the forces which led to the illness: What are the elements of the industrial injury? How did they interact to produce the injury?

It can be recalled from Chapter Two that a stress injury results from two elements—the stressors at work and the susceptibilities of the worker to them. This is presumed to be true because most individuals exposed to a certain stress factor cope with it adequately. Those who don't must have certain vulnerabilities, and these can usually be demonstrated. Understanding of human psychobiology and neurochemistry is incomplete, and the contributions of the two elements cannot always be identified. Also in Chapter Two, there is a discussion of how stress injuries result not from a cause and effect mechanism but from the industrial and non-industrial elements operating together.

First, detailed answers should be obtained about the worker as an individual. The right questions are: What special vulnerabilities did the worker have which contributed to his injury? Is there a major problem in his personal life? How does he ordinarily handle problems? Is his work ethic strong? Is there a history of psychiatric problems or job dissatisfaction?

Secondly, the case manager needs answers about the stressors he faced at work. The right questions are: Was the worker exposed to identifiable job stressors such as overwork, unwanted hours, harassment, a difficult manager, job consolidation, a lack of appreciation, or physical hazards? Is the worker bothered by circumscribed job elements or multiple ones? Are the job conditions he identifies the same ones he had coped with adequately in the past or new ones?

The information obtained about these two elements will show, for instance, that an office worker's panic attacks resulted from an interplay of 1) her histrionic personality and tendency to overreact to stress and 2) the reorganization of her department resulting from a corporate merger. Or it will show that a production supervisor with severe depression accompanying a fractured leg resulted from the interplay of 1) the accident and his subsequent disability and 2) the supervisor's workaholic life style which made him psychologically vulnerable to depression when forced into a period of idleness.

Discovering this interplay is the foundation for creating a dynamic understanding of the stress injury. An accurate understanding of the causative forces will suggest a management strategy which can be applied logically and specifically. The factors which determine the course of the illness are added to this framework one at a time as they are identified by systematic inquiry. An advantage in asking about the elements early is that sometimes no industrial elements can be discovered. It can be shown that the psychiatric disorder claimed by the worker has no connection to his job. The right questions needed to systematically detect these false claims of injury will be introduced later.

The next question for the industrial professional to ask concerns the pitfalls the injured worker may encounter as he moves through the industrial benefit system. These hazards can have real traumatizing effects. They may impede recovery and contribute to health problems which exceed that of the original injury.

The right questions to ask are: Is the system responding adequately to the worker's needs? Are benefits being withheld pending determination of eligibility? Is there still a bond of trust between the injured and the system? How long is the worker expected to remain dependent upon the system?

Having the answers to these questions will sharpen the projection which is slowly forming of the worker's course of recovery. Already, the adjuster or primary care physician may be alerted to noxious influences in the system. An early guess can be made concerning the worker's risks for suffering a psychiatric complication, delayed recovery or excessive disability. This information can be incorporated into the written formulation. Even at this early stage of understanding, steps can be taken to avert these dangers.

At this juncture, knowledge derived from earlier questions about the worker's coping styles can be applied to his involvement in the system. More detailed questions about the worker can be asked: How is this person expected to deal with the rigors of the system? Does he have personality traits which are commonly maladaptive in an industrial system, such as helplessness, psychological immaturity, passive-aggressiveness, paranoia, or a tendency to overreact? Are these the same traits which made him vulnerable to the injury? Are there culturally-determined factors which interfere with his involvement, such as a language barrier, mistrust of authority or lack of familiarity with the system? Does he have an adequate support system?

The dynamic formulation can be enlarged by assessing the worker's psychological reactions to his injury. As outlined in Chapter Four, a person reacts psychologically to his injury in certain normal ways. The most important of these is normal grieving. The four stages of the grief reaction are denial, anger, depression and resolution. Each phase is accompanied by intense emotion which is normal and expected. Such anger and depression are temporary and should not be construed as a discouraging event during a person's recovery. An injury and its associated losses cannot be fully accepted until they are grieved. Persons who fail to go through this reintegrating process are forever immobilized by the shock of the original injury. There are other psychological responses to an injury which are normal and healthy. These include temporary emotional instability, a degree of psychological regression, a reduced ability to handle difficulty, and a spontaneous return to a stable psychological state.

Major physical injuries may be accompanied by excessive anxiety or depression. Occasionally, such workers develop more exotic conditions such as a post-traumatic stress disorder, a phobic aversion or agoraphobia. Frequently, the psychiatric injury persists long after the worker's body has healed, and it is attended by a degree of disability with exceeds that of the physical injury. Similarly, it is important to remember that a person with a psychiatric injury such as a major depression also reacts with his body and mind to the illness. For instance, feeling unstable all the time, being unable to sleep, or feeling terrified of other people, are just as agonizing as an amputation injury or a low back syndrome. A depressed person can feel even more depressed because of this painful mood state, and he can experience aches and pains throughout his body.

The right questions to ask: What are the worker's psychological reactions to his injury? Are they normal or abnormal? Is he adequately grieving his losses?

These questions lead to answers which contribute to the growing understanding of the worker's recuperation as a dynamic process, one which has many interactive influences. Evidence that a worker is reacting abnormally to an injury can be incorporated into the written capsule, alerting the adjuster that recovery will be delayed. Normal grieving will facilitate recovery, and pathological reactions will contribute to complications. Management tactics to prevent these problems can then be initiated. If complications are inevitable, modifications can be made in projecting the outcome of the case.

The next inquiry concerns the issue of secondary gains. This is a critical ingredient in the dynamic formulation of an industrial stress injury, since its presence will totally block treatment, rehabilitation and all other efforts to return the worker to his job. The reasons for this are discussed in detail in Chapter Five. The role of this factor in the effective management of compensation injuries is so important that a clear statement in the formulation about its presence or absence is practically mandatory.

The right questions to ask: Are secondary gain issues present in the case? If not, are there potential ones? Are secondary gain issues expected to enter the case during recovery?

The last question concerns secondary gain behavior which is triggered when a patient feels excessively frustrated during recovery. A common example is a worker who feels unwanted by his employer because he is disabled and who prolongs his recovery to retaliate. This kind of secondary gain behavior might be conceived as a compensation grudge. If a secondary gain mental mechanism is present, the additional question for the consultant is: What is the nature of the secondary gain issue? Detailed answers from the specialist are needed to help the case manager eliminate this obstacle. Until the personal advantages derived from the disability are given up, the energies spent by the system to help the worker will be wasted.

As the consultant ponders these questions, he is looking for reasons that the worker may want to remain ill. Coping with a family problem, needing money, wanting attention, avoiding a noxious work environment, being honorably relieved of an unwanted job, or disguising a weakness are at the top of his list. He wants to identify secondary gain behavior by discovering a current problem such as indebtedness, or an old frustration such as a child with behavioral problems.

A secondary gain mental mechanism should be suspected when a case contains the following elements: delayed healing, an unexplained impasse, treatment failure, a paradoxical response, conflict with an employer or a personal crisis which has a temporal relationship to the accident. References to secondary gains in the doctor's reports are frequently overlooked. Certain lifestyles are associated with a very high incidence of this phenomenon, such as a history of underemployment, poverty, teenage parenting, fraudulent behavior and chemical dependency. Secondary gain issues should be explored in the presence of a problem which might place the worker in a negative light.

To identify secondary gain phenomena, a worker must be examined in the entire context of his personal and occupational life, even areas which are claimed to be free of conflicts. Mention of secondary gains in the written capsule should alert the practitioner that there are serious management problems ahead. If they are deeply-rooted, a poor prognosis is expected.

The next questions concern the treatment conditions faced by the injured worker. The right questions are: Is there a qualified case manager? Has treatment been provided in a timely fashion? Are disruptions expected? Is there sufficient confidentiality? Is the treating doctor familiar with the special factors which influence industrial cases? Is the psychiatric treatment facilitative? Is the treating doctor the same as the evaluating doctor?

Common sense and experience dictate an early diagnosis, timely and appropriate treatment and an emphasis on privacy. Meeting these conditions is ordinarily taken for granted in most health care systems, but in the industrial system, this is a common failing. Too many parties are involved, and the system is slow in responding to the injured worker. Self-interest, fear and litigation pressures shove treatment to the side, and when finally made available, medical intervention is too late or offered in a perfunctory manner.

As discussed in Chapter Six, the conditions for psychiatric treatment are far from optimum. With numerous outside professionals involved and a loss of confidentiality, psychotherapy must be attempted in a "crowded fishbowl." The therapist may not realize that his efforts are being undermined by secondary gain behavior and the manipulation of third and fourth parties. Treatment may be thrown off course by a dynamic formulation which has been made obsolete by a proliferation of determinants which are reinforcing his patient's symptoms. Persons with maladaptive coping styles are overrepresented among these cases, and many are unable to use psychological treatment. Because treatment failure is so common, compensation managers are jaded about authorizing psychotherapy.

The questions asked about treatment conditions require some hard answers. Useless therapy prolongs the worker's exposure to the pitfalls of the industrial system. The adequacy of the treatment setting is incorporated into the written formulation along with the answer to a final question: As a whole, are conditions of treatment sufficiently adequate to justify starting or continuing it?

Management of industrial conditions is greatly distracted by claims of medical conditions which are not compensable. Weeding out false claims of injury can drain the resources of the system and distract from the management of legitimate work conditions. Delays and intensive litigation unfairly penalize those who have a question in their claim. Action on their claim will be suspended, and their numbers contribute to the impression that the natural history of stress injuries is a downhill course. There are good reasons to analyze stress claims early and aggressively, and this is especially true when there are questions concerning the worker's eligibility for industrial benefits. The strategy for diagnosing these pseudoindustrial injuries is the same as that for discovering secondary gain issues. Every area of the worker's functioning, past and present and future, is explored.

The right question to ask: Is there a link between the worker's psychiatric condition and his job?

Malingering, or conscious simulation of injury, is a major distraction in the industrial system. For the claims examiner, it has an elusive nature and is probably the most overly suspected and underdiagnosed condition in his caseload. Its detection is complicated by the absence of any one reliable sign. Certainty about its presence is seldom achieved, but a presumption of malingering is justified when there are multiple positive indicators. The presence of malingering cannot be determined by the absence of objective findings alone. Positive evidence must be identified. It is important to keep in mind that any of these signs may be found in a genuine psychiatric disorder.

A short list of indicators from Chapter Eight includes

a clinical impression that the worker is dissembling, or lying, and that he is observing a caricature of the condition rather than the familiar syndrome. Inconsistencies in the history are noted. There is an impression of missing pieces to the clinical picture. The worker has fraudulent elements in his character or is an antisocial personality. Instinct and clinical experience tell the compensation practitioner he is dealing with a malingerer.

The examiner becomes aware that the individual is highly suggestible, and that he is scrutinizing the examiner for clues which may make a favorable impression. The claimant is vague about his condition at first but talks like an expert as the interview progresses. The psychiatrist observes an abrupt change in the mental status near the end of the interview. The patient looks less disturbed, and the doctor senses he is witnessing the relief that follows a difficult performance. Similarly, the neurologist or orthopedic physician observes changes in the use of a limb when the patient's guard is down. There is an impression that responses to tests of strength or sensation are being altered. Certain accident settings are a positive indicator. These include injuries alleged to have occurred in the parking lot or restroom, or on the first day back to work after a vacation. A high index of suspicion is kept because a relatively minor injury leads to invalid behavior. An easily recognizable personal gain such as money or avoiding responsibility is obvious. When many positive indicators of malingering are found, confirmatory evidence can be obtained from psychological testing or corroborative information.

While determining eligibility, the right questions are: Is the weeding out process being delayed or prolonged? Is it causing a hardship for the claimant? What positive indicators for malingering can be found?

The answers can be incorporated into the dynamic formulation to gain control over this important variable.

This information enables the professional to determine the legitimacy of the claim while minimizing the distracting effects of this process on injury claims which must be accepted as industrial.

Controlling the factors which determine the course of a stress injury must include an assessment of the role played by negative bias. Its presence leads to decisions about psychiatric cases which are based on emotion, a lack of knowledge or traditional prejudice rather than objective information. Too often, a person who suffers a temporary disruption of his psychological equilibrium is looked upon as having something wrong with him which is outside the interest of the medicine. He may be viewed as contemptuous, fraudulent, amoral, or "different" in some nonmedical way. Even the public acceptance of psychiatry as a field of medicine is not strong. Biases about the mentally ill go back for centuries, and they are widespread in contemporary society. Some of the reasons for these attitudes are discussed in Chapter Seven. Their presence in the industrial system causes psychologically-injured workers to be viewed as being unworthy of consideration for its benefits. Underlying this kind of thinking is a tacit denial that psychiatric disorders exist at all.

An attitude of negative bias about stress-related conditions leads to the avoidance of such claimants, and they tend to become the "lepers" of the industrial system. As the issues in their compensation case are neglected, they are at high risk for suffering additional traumas or complications. Managing psychiatric injuries is no different from the management of physical injuries, as each case must be judged on its merits.

It can be seen that negative bias interacts with the element of the worker's enduring personality traits. Injured workers who are characterologically unstable, hostile or overreactive are sometimes viewed as ineligible for benefits because they behave differently from most people. To assure effective management of these claimants, the written formulation must reflect, for instance, that a certain worker is causing the practitioners involved in the case to react negatively. Such counterreactions may lead to management decisions based on emotion or negative bias rather than the facts of the case.

To assess this critical determinant, the right questions are: Is this worker causing people to react to him with intense emotion? Is this case being neglected or undermanaged because it is psychiatric?

The last set of questions involves the early recognition of industrial stress conditions. Timeliness is of major importance in managing stress injuries because the problems created by a delayed diagnosis are so costly. A favorable prognosis depends upon an early understanding of the injury and timely intervention with the right treatment. A systematic way to detect the early signs of psychiatric disorders is offered in Chapter Nine. This chapter contains information about the early manifestations of common stress injuries such as a conversion disorder, somatoform pain disorder, post-traumatic stress disorder, adjustment disorder and organic brain syndrome. Since early recognition depends upon careful monitoring of the course of a worker's recovery, a reminder can be placed at the beginning of the written formulation.

The right question to ask: Is the case being monitored for the early signs of a psychiatric problem?

An abbreviated list from Chapter Nine includes the discovery of delayed healing, unexpected disability in domestic function, and a paradoxical response to treatment. There are early clues in the medical records. The first attending doctors often record their impression that psychological influences are present. There is confusion about the diagnosis as the records contain a long list of diagnoses, or it may be omitted. From the beginning, the case manager is alerted to a psychological crisis which has a temporal relationship with the accident.

Some clues are more subtle and combine with other bits of information, to form a pattern suggesting a psychiatric diagnosis. Examples are excessive use of medication, frequent changes in treatment modality and numerous diagnostic tests or consultations. These prescribed activities suggest the patient is not improving and the doctor is confused. Sameness in the progress reports can be a sign that a physical injury is being influenced by psychological forces. Each report reads like all the others, reflecting an early impasse in the case because of a missed diagnosis or an inaccurate formulation.

Psychiatric injuries often complicate catastrophic accidents such as an explosion, severe chemical exposures, a life-threatening fall, a gunshot wound or an amputation injury. They take the form of a post-traumatic stress disorder or a phobic aversion for reexposing themselves to similar hazards. These conditions can be very debilitating. Anticipation and early detection are of critical importance in preventing chronicity.

The right questions to ask after a major physical injury: Have the treating doctors reported on the patient's psychological reactions to the accident? Are there early signs of a post-traumatic stress disorder or aversion reaction?

Similarly, good management requires an anticipation of complications which occur during the late phases of a worker's recuperation. A plumber with low back syndrome, for instance, may cope with his injury normally until informed by his doctor that he will not improve and has lost his career. At this late stage, the worker has more grieving work to do. He has already lost much time, and this task may be difficult. Another stage to monitor closely is near the end of recovery when a release to work is expected. The patient reports a sudden return of pain and stiffness or a spread of discomfort to other areas. Rather than a setback, these symptoms are psychogenic and reflect the worker's anxieties about going back to work. This can happen when the injury-causing hazard is still present in the work place. Victims of harassment ordinarily experience an increase in their symptoms if they expect to reencounter the offending coworker. In the case of Ms. Allen mentioned earlier in this chapter, fears of confronting the perpetrator at work were so intense that secondary gain issues entered the case early and placed her recovery on hold. In many cases, complications can be anticipated when the doctor is about to send his patient back to work.

The right question to ask: Is a late phase of recovery problem expected?

By asking the right questions, the information obtained from consultants is specific and enables the adjuster and other compensation managers to conceptualize the case soon after the accident. These ideas can be recorded in a synopsis to serve as a reliable guide for creating a management strategy and making decisions during the worker's recovery. If accomplished early, the variables which determine the course of a stress injury can be controlled. Quality management of this kind will counter the natural tendency of psychiatric conditions in industry to have a poor prognosis. Rather than waiting for developments or ignoring the psychiatrically-injured worker, an aggressive and early approach is indicated.

Understanding the dynamics of a psychiatric injury before making major decisions about it will do much to prevent complications. Too many things can go wrong with these conditions from the beginning. To gain control over the determinants, the resources of the system must be expended early, rather than late, in the course of recuperating. Chapter Twelve will elaborate on ways to prevent psychiatric complications.

A willingness to commit to high quality management

of stress injuries will be rewarded by predictability in most cases and an improved prognosis in many. This level of management enables the industrial professional to make optimal use of the system's resources, reduce costs and return the worker to productivity without undue delay. Much of the material of this text is devoted to the reality that many workers cannot adequately utilize its resources, and that shortening their involvement in the system is in everyone's best interest. This caveat leads to three final questions for the compensation practitioner to ask about a case: Is there a willingness to commit to quality management? Is the patient capable of benefitting from it? Is there enough time?

CHAPTER TWELVE

Prevention of Psychiatric Complications

Psychiatric complications are common in an industrial health care system because of its inefficiency and tendency to attract injured people who are unable to handle pressure well. Prevention depends upon providing certain material and intangible services to the injured worker. The tangible ones are self-evident and make up the foundation of every good treatment program. Eligibility is determined quickly along with a diagnosis, and the industrial practitioner obtains enough information to conceptualize the case as a whole. A dynamic formulation and logical management strategy are worked out. Proper treatment is initiated in a timely way, and the injured worker is moving along a path of recovery within a few weeks. If these tasks are not accomplished within this time frame, the worker (or anyone with a medical problem) will begin to feel frustrated.

While these familiar activities are taking place, less tangible tasks must be accomplished. Their influence upon the case is just as important, but they cannot wait even a few weeks. All injured workers have an exquisite sensitivity to the way industrial practitioners are responding to their needs. Right after the injury, the worker is asking himself if anyone cares. He wonders if others are aware of his medical needs or concerned about him as an individual. He wants to learn if he is still important to his employer. He is looking for clues as to how much control he has over his fate, along with the degree of fairness he can expect from the strial system. The intangibles are the attitudes and motives of the people who will help him survive. Genuine interest in the injured worker is the single most crucial ingredient in a good recovery. Within hours or days of the accident, he is capable of detecting the slightest tug of support, interest, neglect or indifference.

The quality of concern by others early-on sets the stage for the worker's future reactions as he moves through the system. First impressions last, and a perception that no one cares will increase his alarm. An injured person feels vulnerable and frightened. Failure to meet needs, both material and emotional, will turn fear into anger. Reactive rage is expressed in perhaps the only way possible for a disabled person, and that is to prolong his recovery. A lack of humanity, withheld treatment or other events which seem unfair to the injured person will increase his risk for having psychiatric complications.

Prevention depends upon treating the worker as an individual with an appreciation of his unique circumstances and a sensitivity to his needs. This is not as difficult as it may seem. Psychiatric complications are usually overdetermined. Multiple frustrations are evidently required to produce these problems. Despite the worker's heightened susceptibility to further injury, he can still deal with minor provocation. Approximate fulfillment of his needs—both material and psychological—may be enough to keep frustrations bearable and facilitate an undelayed recovery. In the service of prevention, a little humanity and concern will go a long way. Unexplained disability can often be traced to the failure to provide the claimant with this critical service.

Pulling through will dominate the mind of the accident victim until he recovers. It is normal to be testing chances for survival at each turn in his case. The first test may involve something seemingly innocuous, such as receiving a telephone call from the employer. Before performing this simple act, an industrial professional should honestly examine his reasons. As described, a disabled person is capable of reading the motives of the people who make decisions about his welfare. A call to express concern will backfire if the real intent is to express irritation or to question the legitimacy of the claim. A call perceived as hostile or showing excessive self-interest can send the worker's recovery on a downhill course.

Some examples which led to complications in actual cases come to mind. A small business owner demanded that his overworked bookkeeper return to her job at once because she was costing him money. A truck driver on leave for anxiety after a collision learned he would be replaced within a week if he didn't show up. A city worker on a leave with back pain was told by personnel that his problem didn't "sound" severe enough to stay at home. In another example, a manager offered unsolicited medical advice over the phone which challenged the doctor's treatment. A medical technician was placed on a three-month medical leave, and the occupational nurse called every week to ask when he might return to his job. One worker decided to consult an outside practitioner when the corporation doctor minimized his shoulder complaints. Two days later, personnel called and accused him of doctor shopping. Infuriated and bewildered, he developed a major depression. Upon reading the chart, I was convinced a caring attitude would have prevented this secondary condition.

The conventional way to respond to an injured acquaintance or coworker is to send a get-well card. This simple token of concern is reassuring, and it does much to create a climate of mutual trust during recuperation. An employer can do even more preventative work by visiting the patient in the hospital and offering assurances about his future employment. Any other opportunity to make a personal contact of a positive nature should be

worker often fails to distinguish between the em-
oyer and the insurance company. He may not be aware his compensation benefits are controlled by someone else. The adjuster can ease the shock of this realization by clarifying things while there is still a bond of trust.

Giving the employee early benefit of the doubt is preventative. A few days' delay in reporting an injury is far more likely to be a result of normal denial of serious injury than a late fabrication. The fact that only a single worker out of dozens subjected to a stressor files a claim of injury suggests a psychological vulnerability more than it does an act of malingering.

Giving the benefit of the doubt is especially important when making telephone contact. If a child answers the telephone and says his parent isn't home, the urge to ask his whereabouts must be restrained. This particular indiscretion is a recurring complaint among workers who later developed a compensation grudge. Being on a medical leave doesn't mean a worker must stay at home. If information is volunteered that a disabled employee is shopping, doing volunteer work or visiting out-of-state relatives, it doesn't mean he is abusing his benefits. Part of the adjuster's job (or anyone's job in the compensation field) is confronting an irate claimant over the telephone. While such anger at first may seem unreasonable, it may not be, and hearing out an upset employee can be preventative. The listener, for instance, may be the first to learn of a major threat to the worker's recovery. Perhaps the most neglected opportunity to prevent psychiatric complications is making supportive contact with a worker who is physically injured in an accident which becomes the subject of a safety investigation. While accountability pressures cause everyone involved to feel stressed, they are especially hard on the worker who is the least able to defend himself and usually the last to learn of his role in the accident. In this situation the employee tends to feel isolated and abandoned. The mental anguish during the investigation may greatly exceed the pain of the physical injury. Supportive contact can be preventative after any accident when there are pressures to find a scapegoat. A firm can do much to preserve its human resources by making certain that an injured employee receives positive responses both early and throughout his recovery.

Self-insured corporations and municipalities with in-house adjusters are in the best position to prevent secondary stress disorders as services can be coordinated. Teamwork can meet a worker's needs more efficiently and gain a firmer control of the determinants which shape his recovery. Large employers use two of the best preventative strategies applied thus far in industry. The first concerns modifying the job setting so an injured worker may return to work as soon as possible. Removing a noxious co-worker, transferring the worker to a different department, distributing a work load more fairly or offering more reasonable hours, as examples, are excellent ways to keep disability to an irreducible minimum. In the case of a physical injury, the dilemma of "no light work" can be prevented, and work-hardening programs can be employed. Because of their considerable resources, self-insureds run a higher risk of conflict of interest problems. Departments providing liaison services have a job requiring much tact, and they cannot be expected to make everyone happy. Keeping a careful eye on activities which imperil the worker's recovery may be greatly preventative. It is hard to imagine a reason for showing indignance when an employee informs the occupational medicine department he wants to have a private physician. And it is expected that most workers would be hurt by actions taken by the personnel department, for example, which are unfairly self-serving.

The second proven preventative measure available to large employers is free counseling sessions for workers who feel stressed by their job. Treatment is self-directed and unencumbered by the issues which must be settled in a preauthorized scheme. These programs provide the earliest possible intervention for people in very stressful occupations, such as police officers, firemen, emergency dispatchers, correctional officers and social service workers. Emotional distress caused by day-to-day work demands is reduced before it escalates into a full-blown stress injury such as depression or "burnout." Because of their accessibility, these programs can prevent the complications arising from physical injuries. All employers could reduce the disability from stress by providing this service.

The doctor responding to the stressed worker can do much preventative work by being less eager to order a disability leave. While his patient may experience relief when removed from a noxious job, valuable time and opportunities are lost in remedying a problem which still must be faced when his release is signed. Regardless of how upset the worker is, a medical leave is not always mandatory. This action places his patient in the industrial health care system, which may not resolve his patient's dilemma. More often than not, it aggravates the problem. Once on disability, the employee undergoes a drastic change in the way he is viewed by his company. He is labelled an "injured worker," and this sets in motion a series of departmental involvements and medical assessments which are required by policy. These activities place him at risk for acquiring another label—a "problem employee." A common result is an irreversible adversary relationship with his company.

Many job crises can be resolved by the worker if he is encouraged to use his own initiative, such as approaching his manager or opening up channels of assistance created by the company for this purpose. This is best done before his employer is forced to treat him as an injured or troubled worker. The doctor practices preventative medicine when he discusses these alternatives with his patient. As pointed out in Chapter Nine on facilitative treatment, "no treatment" is often a good alternative in the industrial system. More than any other "therapy," it promotes self-sufficiency and tailor-made solutions. It may be especially preventative with workers who typically cope with job stress by acting helpless. The doctor who is quick to order a disability leave often finds himself with a patient who expects his leave to be extended repeatedly. Here, the worker's helplessness is reinforced rather than confronted, and his physician contributes to a preventable disability. As indicated above, the end result is often a broken bond of trust with his employer and a lost job. Before placing his job-stressed patient on a medical leave, the attending doctor must assess the risk/benefit aspects of his decision.

The attorney is also in a position to do preventative work. His expertise can be applied by shortening the injured worker's stay in the industrial system. As pointed out before in this text, many injured people lack the capacity for making constructive use of their treatment and rehabilitation benefits. Their inflexibility and precarious emotional stability do not stand up well to the frustrations encountered in a multi-party health care system. They are at high risk for being overwhelmed and for developing psychiatric complications. In this situation, a risk/benefit dilemma also faces the attorney. Repeated attempts to obtain these benefits must be weighed against the harm done in the form of prolonged dependency upon the system and predictably, increased suffering and disability. Like the other players in the system, the attorney must recognize that his most helpless-appearing claimant has more resources than he claims. To an extent not ordinarily appreciated, the helpless worker is trying to manipulate someone else into taking over his problem. By assuming too much responsibility for his client's welfare, the attorney paradoxically places him in an even more needy and helpless position.

As outlined in Chapter Eleven, the adjuster can prevent complications by using his consultants early rather than later. The information from professionals can be used to accurately conceptualize the case, and more importantly, gain early control over the determinants which shape recovery. With specific answers to his questions, the adjuster can identify those claimants who are unable to make effective use of their benefits and reduce the time they are exposed to the hazards of the system. Quality management of this sort will be rewarded by an improved prognosis in many cases. With prevention in mind, he can once again ask himself the questions: Am I interested in a quality management? Can the injured worker benefit from it? Is there time?

Industrial Stress Injuries may suggest what policy makers can do to facilitate an undelayed recovery for the injured worker (or to otherwise improve the efficiency of the industrial health care system). Several ideas come to mind for the top of the list: There is access to a certain number of self-directed counseling sessions for the stressed worker. A greater emphasis is placed on modifying the injured worker's environment. There is more education for industrial practitioners, including physicians who treat injured workers, about the interplay of determinants which control the course of these injuries. Also on such a list is an earlier use of consultants to promote a better understanding of the worker. This knowledge will enable the system to respond to him in an timely and individualized way. Lastly, there is a way to monitor the worker's progress to protect him from an excessive exposure to the system.

References

References

Alexander, F. (1950). *Psychosomatic medicine: its principles and applications.* New York: W.W. Norton.

Anthony, N. (1976). Malingering as role-taking. *Journal of Clinical Psychology, 32,* 32-41.

Boxer, P.A. (1984). An epidemic of psychogenic illness in an electronics plant. *J Occup Med, 26,* 381-385.

Bromberg, W. (1979). Functional overlay: an illegitimate diagnosis? *West J Med, 130,* 561-565.

Bursten, B. (1986). Psychiatric injury in women's workplaces. *Bull Am Acad Psychiatry Law, 14,* 245-251.

Casella, C. (1986). Public acceptance of psychiatry. *Psychiatric Times,* April, 1986.

Chodoff, P. (1978). Psychiatry and the fiscal third party. *Am J Psychiatry, 135,* 1141-1147.

Crull P. (1982). Stress effects of sexual harassment on the job: implications for counseling. *Am J Orthopsychiatry 52,* 539-544, 1982.

Davis, J. (1985). Workers' compensation claims for stress-related disorders. *J Occup Med, 27,* 821-825.

Derebery, V.J., Tullis, W.H. (1983). Delayed recovery in the patient with a work compensable injury. *J Occup Med 25,* 829-835.

Diagnostic and Statistical Manual of Mental Disorders (Third Edition-Revised) (1987). American Psychiatric Association.

Diamond, B. (1959). The fallacy of the impartial expert. *Archives of Criminal Psychodynamics 3,* 221-236.

Dworkin, R.H., Handlin, D.S. (1985). Unraveling the effects of compensation, litigation and employment on treatment of chronic pain. *Pain 23,* 49-59.

Fenichel, O. (1945). *The psychoanalytical theory of neurosis.* New York: W.W. Norton & Company.

Freud, S. (1963). *General introduction to psychoanalysis.* New York: Washington Square Press.

Freud, S. (1955). *Mourning and melancholia, standard edition of the complete psychological works of Sigmund Freud, Vol 14.* Hogarth Press.

Fromm-Reichmann, F. (1950). *Principles of intensive psychotherapy.* University of Chicago Press.

Goldney, R.D. (1984). Elucidation of psychological factors in compensable injury. *Med J Aust 141,* 433-436.

Goldsmith, F. (1982). *Occupational safety and health.* New York: Human Sciences Health.

Green, S.A. (1985). *Mind and body: the psychology of physical illness.* Washington, DC: American Psychiatric Press.

Greenson, R. (1971). *The technique and practice of psychoanalysis.* New York: International Universities Press.

Halleck, S.L. (1971). *The politics of therapy.* New York: Science House.

Hirschfeld, A.H., Behan, R.C. (1963). The accident process 1: Etiological considerations of industrial injuries. *JAMA 186,* 193-199.

Hirschfeld, A.H., Behan, R.C. (1963). The accident process II: toward more rational treatment of industrial injuries. *JAMA 186,* 300-306.

Hirshfeld, A.H., Behan, R.C. (1966). The accident process. *JAMA 197,* 85-89.

Keir, H.J. (1987). *Textbook of occupational medicine.* New York: Churchill Livingstone.

Kuiper, P.C. (1967). *On being genuine.* New York: Basic Books.

Kurtz, P. (1989). A variant of mass (epidemic) psychogenic illness in an agricultural work setting. *J Occup Med 31,* 331-334.

Leavitt, F. (1987). Detection of simulation among persons instructed to exaggerate symptoms of low back pain. *J Occup Med 29,* 229-233.

Levenson, H. (1980). Industrial accidents and recent life events. *J Occup Med 22,* 53-57.

Levenson, H., Hirschfeld, M.L. (1983). Recent life events and accidents: the role of sex differences. *Journal of Human Stress,* March 1983, 4-11.

Maslach, C. (1982). *Burnout—the cost of caring.* Englewood Cliffs, New Jersey: Prentice-Hall.

Mendelson, G. (1983). The effects of compensaton and litigation on disability following compensable injuries. *Am J Forensic Psychiatry 4,* 97-112.

Menninger, K. (1959). *A psychiatrist's world.* New York: Viking Press.

Menninger, K. (1963). *The vital balance.* New York: Viking Press.

Menninger, W.C. (1947). Psychosomatic medicine: somatization reactions. *Psychosom Med, 9,* 92-97.

Menninger, W.C. (1967). *A psychiatrist for a troubled world* New York: Viking Press.

Meyer, A. (1957). *Psychobiology: a science of man.* Springfield, Illinois: Charles C. Thomas.

Modlin, H.C. (1986). Compensation Neurosis. *Bull Am Acad Psychiatry Law 14,* 263-271.

Morris, L.E. (1970). Over the hump in Vietnam: adjustment patterns in a time-limited stress situation. *Bull Menninger Clinic, 34,* 352-362.

Nemiah, J.C. (1978). The dynamic bases of psychopathology, in (Nicholi, A., ed.) *The Harvard guide to modern psychiatry.* Cambridge: The Belknap Press of Harvard University Press.

Parad, H. (1965). *Crisis intervention.* New York: Family Services Association of America.

Parker, N. (1977). Accident litigants with neurotic symptoms. *Med J Aust, 2,* 318-322.

Rutter, M. (1986). Meyerian psychobiology, personality development and the role of life experiences. *Am J Psychiatry 143,* 1077-1087.

Rutter, M. (1985). Resilience in the face of adversary: protective factors and resistance to psychiatric disorders. *Br J Psychiatry, 147,* 598-611.

Tager, R.M. (1985). Simulated disability. *J Occup Med, 27,* 915-916.

Sander, R.A. (1986). The relationship of disability to compensation status in railroad workers. *Spine, 11,* 141-143.

Zenz, B.S. (1983). *Occupational Health.* Boston: Little Brown.